IT HAPPENED TO ME

Series Editor: Arlene Hirschfelder

Books in the It Happened to Me series are designed for inquisitive teens digging for answers about certain illnesses, social issues, or lifestyle interests. Whether you are deep into your teen years or just entering them, these books are gold mines of up-to-date information, riveting teen views, and great visuals to help you figure out stuff. Besides special boxes highlighting singular facts, each book is enhanced with the latest reading lists, websites, and an index. Perfect for browsing, there are loads of expert information by acclaimed writers to help parents, guardians, and librarians understand teen illness, tough situations, and lifestyle choices.

1. *Epilepsy: The Ultimate Teen Guide,* by Kathlyn Gay and Sean McGarrahan, 2002.
2. *Stress Relief: The Ultimate Teen Guide,* by Mark Powell, 2002.
3. *Learning Disabilities: The Ultimate Teen Guide,* by Penny Hutchins Paquette and Cheryl Gerson Tuttle, 2003.
4. *Making Sexual Decisions: The Ultimate Teen Guide,* by L. Kris Gowen, 2003.
5. *Asthma: The Ultimate Teen Guide,* by Penny Hutchins Paquette, 2003.
6. *Cultural Diversity—Conflicts and Challenges: The Ultimate Teen Guide,* by Kathlyn Gay, 2003.
7. *Diabetes: The Ultimate Teen Guide,* by Katherine J. Moran, 2004.
8. *When Will I Stop Hurting? Teens, Loss, and Grief: The Ultimate Teen Guide to Dealing with Grief,* by Ed Myers, 2004.
9. *Volunteering: The Ultimate Teen Guide,* by Kathlyn Gay, 2004.
10. *Organ Transplants—A Survival Guide for the Entire Family: The Ultimate Teen Guide,* by Tina P. Schwartz, 2005.
11. *Medications: The Ultimate Teen Guide,* by Cheryl Gerson Tuttle, 2005.
12. *Image and Identity—Becoming the Person You Are: The Ultimate Teen Guide,* by L. Kris Gowen and Molly C. McKenna, 2005.
13. *Apprenticeship: The Ultimate Teen Guide,* by Penny Hutchins Paquette, 2005.
14. *Cystic Fibrosis: The Ultimate Teen Guide,* by Melanie Ann Apel, 2006.
15. *Religion and Spirituality in America: The Ultimate Teen Guide,* by Kathlyn Gay, 2006.
16. *Gender Identity: The Ultimate Teen Guide,* by Cynthia L. Winfield, 2007.

17. *Physical Disabilities: The Ultimate Teen Guide,* by Denise Thornton, 2007.
18. *Money—Getting It, Using It, and Avoiding the Traps: The Ultimate Teen Guide,* by Robin F. Brancato, 2007.
19. *Self-Advocacy: The Ultimate Teen Guide,* by Cheryl Gerson Tuttle and JoAnn Augeri Silva, 2007.
20. *Adopted: The Ultimate Teen Guide,* by Suzanne Buckingham Slade, 2007.
21. *The Military and Teens: The Ultimate Teen Guide,* by Kathlyn Gay, 2008.
22. *Animals and Teens: The Ultimate Teen Guide,* by Gail Green, 2009.
23. *Reaching Your Goals: The Ultimate Teen Guide,* by Anne Courtright, 2009.
24. *Juvenile Arthritis: The Ultimate Teen Guide,* by Kelly Rouba, 2009.
25. *Obsessive-Compulsive Disorder: The Ultimate Teen Guide,* by Natalie Rompella, 2009.
26. *Body Image and Appearance: The Ultimate Teen Guide,* by Kathlyn Gay, 2009.
27. *Writing and Publishing: The Ultimate Teen Guide,* by Tina P. Schwartz, 2010.
28. *Food Choices: The Ultimate Teen Guide,* by Robin F. Brancato, 2010.
29. *Immigration: The Ultimate Teen Guide,* by Tatyana Kleyn, 2011.
30. *Living with Cancer: The Ultimate Teen Guide,* by Denise Thornton, 2011.
31. *Living Green: The Ultimate Teen Guide,* by Kathlyn Gay, 2012.
32. *Social Networking: The Ultimate Teen Guide,* by Jenna Obee, 2012.
33. *Sports: The Ultimate Teen Guide,* by Gail Fay, 2013.
34. *Adopted: The Ultimate Teen Guide, Revised Edition,* by Suzanne Buckingham Slade, 2013.
35. *Bigotry and Intolerance: The Ultimate Teen Guide,* by Kathlyn Gay, 2013.
36. *Substance Abuse: The Ultimate Teen Guide,* by Sheri Bestor, 2013.
37. *LGBTQ Families: The Ultimate Teen Guide,* by Eva Apelqvist, 2013.
38. *Bullying: The Ultimate Teen Guide,* by Mathangi Subramanian, 2014.
39. *Eating Disorders: The Ultimate Teen Guide,* by Jessica R. Greene, 2014.
40. *Speech and Language Challenges: The Ultimate Teen Guide,* by Marlene Targ Brill, 2014.
41. *Divorce: The Ultimate Teen Guide,* by Kathlyn Gay, 2014.

SPEECH AND LANGUAGE CHALLENGES

THE ULTIMATE TEEN GUIDE

MARLENE TARG BRILL

IT HAPPENED TO ME, NO. 40

ROWMAN & LITTLEFIELD

Lanham • Boulder • New York • Toronto • London

Published by Rowman & Littlefield
4501 Forbes Boulevard, Suite 200, Lanham, Maryland 20706
www.rowman.com

16 Carlisle Street, London W1D 3 BT, United Kingdom

British Library Cataloguing in Publication Information Available

Library of Congress Cataloging-in-Publication Data

Brill, Marlene Targ.
  Speech and language challenges : the ultimate teen guide / Marlene Targ Brill.
    pages cm. — (It happened to me ; no. 40)
  Audience: Grades 9-12.
  Includes bibliographical references and index.
  ISBN 978-0-8108-8791-6 (cloth : alk. paper) — ISBN 978-0-8108-8792-3 (ebook)
  1. Communicative disorders in adolescence. I. Title.
  RJ496.C67B75 2014
  616.85'88900835—dc23   2014007973

Contents

Acknowledgments vii

Introduction: Let's Talk Speech and Language ix

1 The Amazing Story of Communication 1

2 When Words Won't Flow: Stuttering and
Other Fluency Challenges 15

3 Mixed-Up Sounds and Words: Speech Sound Disorders 41

4 When the Voice Goes Haywire: Voice Disorders 59

5 When the Brain Hears and Processes Information Differently:
Language Disorders 75

6 Cars, Guns, Sports, and the Unexpected: Brain Injury and
Communication 105

7 When English Is New or Sounds Different 129

8 Technology as a Communication Game Changer 155

9 Looking Ahead: Boosting Communications Skills All Around 183

Glossary 207

Notes 211

Index 223

About the Author 229

Acknowledgments

I like to think that this book is mine—or at least all my doing. But that is definitely not true. Publishing a book takes a community, one that ranges from assistance with content ideas and research through interviews and checking facts and editing. This was the case with *Speech and Language Challenges*. Without the following people, this book would not exist.

I cannot thank enough the brave teens and adults who shared their stories. Some interviewees are still finding their way with communication challenges. Others have achieved peace with their speech and languages differences and have overcome difficulties that were once definitely problematic. The thoughtful insights shared in their stories will help other teens along their communication journey. I especially want to acknowledge Katherine Guardado, Stuart Kaufman, Rachel Neuses, Susannah Parkin, Roxanne Swentzell, and Shannon Thomas for their courage and suggestions. Visuals from Shane Garcia, Temple Grandin, Stuart Kaufman, Anne Ryan, Roxanne Swentzell, and supportive organizations such as the Stuttering Foundation and We Stop Hate add to these stories. Any success with this book comes from these strong and persevering individuals.

A book with technical information, such as this one, depends upon the kindness of knowledgeable professionals. Hearty thanks to these experts in their fields: speech and language pathologists Sue Cantor, Christy Cook, Iris Gimbel, Joanne Hein, Suzi Shulman, and Erman Vandy; audiologists Malvina Levy and Karena Weil; and educational specialists Arlene Erlbach and Lucy Klocksin. I received assistance locating interviewees from Rozanne Clauson, American Speech-Language-Hearing Association, and Scot Squires, the Stuttering Foundation. Both organizations are top resources in their fields. Further, I want to thank Richard Brill for his computer technical expertise in formatting this book, and Alison Brill, public health consultant, Suzi Shulman, and my amazing editor, Arlene Hirschfelder, for their guidance and critical review of the manuscript. Any remaining mistakes are all mine.

Introduction:
Let's Talk Speech and Language

Like most people, you might figure you should be able to take talking for granted. When you want to say something, well, you just say it. On the flip side, you assume someone nearby will listen and respond when you talk. Not so easy for everyone.

For some teens, communicating can be a chore. They find their words spill out at an uneven rate. Or they say or hear words differently. Any number of problems talking, listening, and communicating can occur. Simple conversation becomes so frustrating that it turns into a source of stress.

What do teens do? In extreme situations, they choose not to talk at all. In others, such as when saying the letter *r* or stuttering is the problem, they say words they can pronounce easily. Both options can be limiting. Way too often, this restricting of communications causes problems at school, work, or with friends.

Why Read This Book?

This book tackles some of the varied issues teens experience with speech and language difficulties. Equally important, the content offers suggestions that may ease these challenges. Personal stories help readers understand the impact of a communication challenge. These examples and explanations inform those who have or know someone who has a communication difficulty. In addition, the text provides information for those who find the topics interesting and want to know more, whether for a report or general knowledge. A glossary at the end lists key terms and their definitions.

The idea of writing about communication challenges arose after investigation uncovered that no comprehensive book exists for adolescents about the topic. Sure there are books about individual subjects mentioned in the chapters, such as stuttering or auditory processing difficulties caused by serious head injury. But no book tackles the many types of communication issues that can occur. And no title expands the definition of communication to include differences caused by learning English as a second language or difficulties resulting from reliance on technology. Even if you do not have a specific communication challenge, you may confront these serious areas as your world enlarges beyond the local community.

Once research accumulated for this book, the breadth of topics involved with speech, language, and hearing expanded. With more in-depth research, I confirmed that these topics needed to be included. Hopefully, you will find them helpful and interesting, too.

Who Has a Communication Problem?

According to the U.S. Department of Education 2010 report to Congress, 3 of every 100 students ages three to twenty-one receive school services for speech and language problems.[1] Of the 6.1 million children with disabilities who obtain special education services in public schools, more than 1.1 million participate in speech and language therapy.[2] Nearly 50 million Americans experience a speech, language, or hearing disorder.

If these figures are not enough, consider that 10 percent of the world's population encounters conditions that interfere with normal communication some time in their lives. Stuttering alone accounts for 3 million people of all ages in the United States and 67 million people worldwide.[3] For all these people, a problem

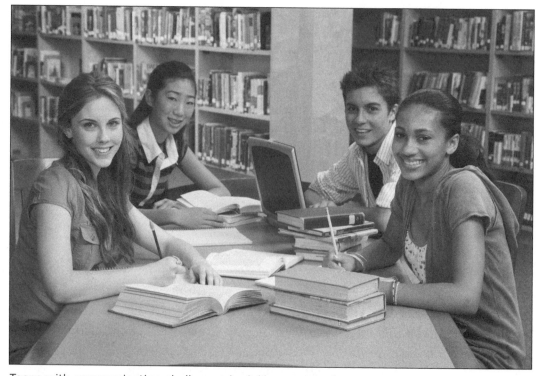

Teens with communication challenges look like anyone else.

with communicating affects every aspect of their lives. School, dating, social life, work—it all depends upon how someone communicates.

Speech, language, and hearing challenges cross gender and racial lines. Boys or girls from any community can find they have trouble talking, listening, and communicating. So you—or anyone you know with a speech problem—are not alone.

What seems like effortless speech to some is really a complex process involving messages to and from the brain, muscle movements, and timing. Many factors can interfere with the success of these interactions. Perhaps reduced hearing poses a problem, causing difficulty understanding incoming messages. Or the brain can't relay messages correctly to and from speech centers. In some cases, forming a response proves impossible, either because the brain distorts messages or the motor mechanism to respond is damaged. With other cases, teens may lack experiences to adapt language to different situations. Any of these scenarios can be embarrassing and troublesome.

What Does a Speech Problem Look Like?

In a weird way, another problem for teens with speech challenges is how the person looks. People who have other physical disabilities look a certain way. They may use a wheelchair or crutches, or display irregular characteristics or movements. Anyone with a communication challenge, however, usually looks like nothing is wrong—at least until starting to talk. Certain expectations arise because the individual appears "regular." When these expectations aren't met, such as sounds not fitting the look of the person, there is a disconnect for the listener. Communication stalls, if it happens at all. Dating, responding in class or on the job, making friends. All these areas suffer, sometimes turning into awkward situations for speakers and listeners.

This book explores how regular speech develops, and then investigates which challenges occur, how they happen, and what can be done to ease speech and language differences. You will discover what it means to have fluency, voice, articulation, or brain trauma disorders. You will explore experiences a newcomer has grappling with a foreign language and how technology is changing how everyone communicates.

Eliminating Myths

A key objective of the book is to dispel myths about teens who experience communication challenges. Another goal is to build understanding—for the teen with

> "I grew up with a stutter, acutely afraid of trying to get through simple sentences, knowing that I would then, or later, be the subject of ridicule."
> —Vice President Joe Biden[a]

a speech and language disorder and for friends and family—in order to help everyone get along better.

One reality that interferes with such harmony involves mistaken assumptions about someone who has a speech or language problem. Sadly, too many myths exist. Time to get real. Here are ten common myths about people who talk differently that are plain fantasy:

1. People with speech problems are less intelligent or capable than those who produce regular speech. Nothing could be further from the truth. Trouble speaking, without an accompanying mental, emotional, or developmental disability, has little connection to brain power, competence, or future success. In this book, you'll read about teens with speech disorders who have become successful in many varied fields.

2. Speech problems, such as stuttering, can be controlled, if only someone has the will. Not so. Speech disorders develop from a variety of causes, such as motor coordination problems or brain trauma. Therapy helps teens deal with these issues and progress, but such problems are not mere habits that can be broken simply by choice and will power.

3. Speech problems indicate mental disorder. Speech and language issues are never predictors of mental instability. However, constant teasing or bullying because of a speech disorder may trigger emotional responses, and these may have an impact on mental disorders.

4. Speech and language problems are caused by bad parenting. As a teen, you may assume your parents contribute to all your problems. But be assured that a speech or language disorder is not one of them. In fact, parents can be your best advocate. Who else can help find a therapist or deal with school administrators who refuse to provide necessary therapy or classroom support? And who else will lend a supportive ear when communication interferes with your other relationships?

5. Once teens have a speech disorder, they will always experience problems. Therapists and activities they suggest can help teens improve language and communication skills. In fact, some teens progress to the point that the problem becomes unnoticeable. Even if some disorders, such as stuttering, last a lifetime, they don't have to remain a disability.

6. Speech and language disorders happen only in young kids. Many speech problems begin when language develops or does not progress. But others can develop at any age. Car accidents. Sports injuries to the head. Strokes, those pesky blood clots that travel to the brain. Any of these traumas can damage parts of the brain that control input and output of messages.

7. *Growing up in a bilingual home contributes to speech disorders.* Sometimes, teens from bilingual homes switch from one language to another to find the perfect word. But this is not a speech problem. Knowing another language is a plus. Coming from another country during preteen or teen years can be troublesome, however, until someone learns enough new words and grammar to communicate effectively. Immigrant teens must also learn different customs concerning when certain language applies. But such accommodations are not considered a disorder. Most can be corrected with time, direction, and practice.

8. *People get speech problems from emotional traumas.* It's true that traumatic events can trigger an inability to talk clearly. In fact, some people who stutter began stuttering after such an episode. But in these situations, usually regular speech and language may return once sporadic emotional factors subside. Those challenges that do not go away come from an inborn tendency toward the problem that was sparked by trauma. These situations will be explored later in this book.

9. *People with speech issues are more nervous and shy.* Certainly, when teens become self-conscious about feeling different in any area of their lives, they may lose confidence. This loss can appear as nervousness or shyness. But once people who have trouble speaking learn to deal with their disorder, they experience the same range of emotions as other teens.

10. *There is nothing anyone can do for a friend or relative who has a speech problem.* If someone you know has a speech problem, there are several dos and don'ts that contribute to smoothing communication. Read on to learn answers to your questions about speech disorders and how you can help someone who has difficulty speaking.

THE AMAZING STORY OF COMMUNICATION

Communication is one of the most remarkable human achievements. The idea that as a tiny baby you develop the facility to use words, symbols, and gestures to acquire and transmit information is astounding. Speech, or oral language, involves a series of complex movements that allow you to produce specific sounds. Coordinated muscles in your head, neck, chest, and abdomen actually produce the sounds.

With such complicated processes, difficulties are bound to occur. Estimates are that between 6 and 8 million people in the United States deal with some form of issue producing language. To better define and address speech and language challenges, it helps to understand how you acquire these skills. Only then can you recognize the range of normal development and what can go wrong.

Learning Language

Communication begins with a cry. Crying helps babies alert parents to their needs. Infants also tense their body or flail arms and legs. They turn red. As time passes, infants cry less and define their movements better. At the same time, they produce more sounds, inching toward saying words and gaining greater control over their social environment.

Babies first learn to communicate by observing language. When able, they try to imitate what they see and hear. They practice vowel and consonant sounds representative of language around them. For example, in English-speaking families, babies notice and try to reproduce sounds that form the English language. In France, babies try to reproduce the same French sounds their caretakers say. Slowly, these sounds turn into letters, words, and sentences.

Communication is transmitted by means of two main pathways. Receptive language involves understanding words, symbols, and gestures. Mainly, it's the information you take in. Expressive language is the ability to relate information through these same avenues, which is how you use language. Expressive language is the information that is shared. Most children understand (receptive) more than they are able to communicate (expressive).

Many people assume that speech and language refer to the same thing. It's true that both help teens communicate and share thoughts, ideas, and emotions. But there are some key differences. *Speech* refers to how sounds are produced, or the mechanism of generating language. *Language* is what you say and when. Essentially, this is how communication occurs in various social situations.

Talking about Language

The words and how they are put together to convey messages involve a set of communication rules. These rules may differ, depending upon the social group—race, religion, nationality, community—that shares them. Different cultures have guidelines for expressing messages. Some communications within a given culture are acceptable in one social situation but not in another.

A family in the United States may use language that is different and in different settings than families from the Middle East or Mexico. In the United States, for example, teens never use two forms of *the* to indicate whether a word is male or female. Only specific humans and other animals warrant that gender distinction. But people who speak Spanish use *la* or *el* when referring to words they identify as female or male. Most often, the words are nouns, such as the names of people. But many are objects, such as *la carta* (letter) or *el libro* (book). In English speakers merely say (the) letter or book.

Rules from varying social groups govern how every participant in that group exchanges their thoughts. People from each group might address strangers or family members in more or less formal ways. Similarly, some settings require more casual or more formal language. For example, what you say and how you

---

❗ Tim's Awesome Language Skills

Tim Doner, age seventeen, is known as a hyper-polyglot teen. How did he get that label? By learning twenty languages. Polyglot is the Greek term for "many languages." The *hyper* prefix indicates that he speaks more than four languages fluently: French, Arabic, Hebrew, Farsi, Chinese, German, and Russian.

"I feel language gives you a way to connect with another person," Doner said. "Each language is in many ways an expression of how one society or culture thinks. I feel that when I start to speak foreign languages, a lot of times I become a bit of a different person."[a]

What Do You Say?

Researcher and doctoral student Joshua Katz at North Carolina State University, surveyed what people in different parts of the United States called the same thing.[b]

He found some funny differences. Did you know that easterners say "soda," midwesterners say "pop," and southerners specify "coke," while westerners just say "soft drink"—all for the same fizzy drink? Or have you considered that how you address a group of people depends on where you live? "Y'all" is very southern, "you all" is western," and "you guys" is northwestern. Who knew?

express yourself during a job interview is different, or should be, from how you talk at home or school with friends and family. You might even tell one parent something you wouldn't dare share with the other. In these and similar cases, communications within a culture can be dictated by location or setting.

Language consists of learning these varied meanings for words. In turn, English speakers can take certain base words and turn them into new words with slightly different meanings. A good example is *happy*, *happier*, or *unhappy*.

Once teens learn certain base words, they can arrange them with other words in a specific order that expresses what they are thinking. If you said, "Dance Jane you will me with," someone might understand that the speaker really means, "Jane, will you dance with me?" But the second version will probably be much easier for English speakers to understand. And the desired response would come quicker than with the first attempt.

Language can also be expressed in ways other than by speaking. Someone can write—including handwriting, e-mail, texting, or tweeting—sign with their fingers, or use other body language. Some people with neurological disorders may communicate through eye blinks or head or mouth movements. Each form of expression has its own standards.

Talking about Speech

Speech is one form of language that focuses on how you talk, or communicate verbally. It requires a miraculous combination of timing, nerve messages, and muscle control. Verbal communication follows its own set of rules. Speech involves word formation, which includes sounds put together to form words. Speech also covers word production, or what comes out of your mouth. Speakers form these words so others can hear and understand them. This, too, is part of communicating language. Voices may be shrill or bell-like in tone; they may be blasting or a whisper in volume. All these differences fall within a typical range of speaking.

Speech consists of several elements, which will be explored in more detail in other chapters. Articulation incorporates how speech sounds are expressed. For example, children learn to form words beginning with *r* so they can say "rabbit" rather than "wabbit," which they might say at a younger age. How and if sounds are produced, such as whether you are hoarse or lose your voice altogether, involves *voice*. The rhythm of word flow is affected by fluency. These elements, plus

Babies and the Miracle of Speaking

All babies begin life with the same range of sounds. They babble and coo and sputter blueberries, which usually causes onlookers to laugh. How do these interesting sounds turn into understandable language? By caretakers, which includes those of you who babysit, repeating sounds they want the baby to ultimately learn. Caretakers make up sound games or smile when babies produce certain sounds. In this way, caretakers reinforce particular sounds that make up their particular language. Over time, this reinforcement directs babies to retain and repeat specific sounds while allowing others to fall away. The result is babies eventually learn to put sounds together that form words in the family's language. Those of you who have younger siblings probably observed this already.

Similarly, people from the same country can learn different accents. This, too, depends upon which sounds are reinforced in young children—and a good ear for sounds. People from one part of the United States may have different inflections, or ways of saying certain sounds, from those in other parts of the country. Think how someone with a Southern drawl sounds when compared with Midwest nasal tones. What about the difference in English between British singer Adele and Texas-born actor Matthew McConaughey? Sometimes, you pick up an accent after spending considerable time in a place where people speak differently. That's all part of learning and reinforcement that gives you new skills throughout a lifetime.

general understanding of language and perceiving messages of others, influence speech and language development.

Developing Typical Patterns

Children display a broad range of abilities to speak and understand what they hear. They mature through a continual process that combines inborn abilities with information from the world around them. Both speech and language develop in specific regular steps. Each accomplishment lays the groundwork for the next. Basic skills grow more complex with experience. This exciting process is called development. Educators and doctors examine these developmental steps at certain intervals to ensure children are maturing in a typical manner. They call the steps milestones (see table 1.1).

Within each milestone, however, individuals develop through a range of speeds and abilities that are completely normal. Some children progress quickly as they mature, while others seem slower. Still others may follow a pattern of fits

Table 1.1. Amazing Communication Milestones[1]

	Speech	Language
Newborns	Cries; makes pleasure sounds, such as cooing	Reacts to loud sounds; sucks in response to sounds
By six months	Babbles in different sounds, beginning with *p*, *m*; makes noises when played with; gurgles when playing alone; imitates sounds and syllables; vocalizes, chuckles, laughs	Looks in direction of sounds; tries to communicate with actions; indicates pleasure and displeasure; looks toward sounds, music
By twelve months	Babbles ("ba-ba," "ma-ma"); says two or three words; recognizes words for items	Points to picture/object when named; listens when others speak; uses gestures to communicate; waves bye-bye

(continued)

Table 1.1. (*continued*)

	Speech	Language
By two years	Says about fifty words in two- to four-word sentences; names body parts, familiar people/ hard to understand	Follows simple directions; points to things in books or pictures; understands about 300 words
By three years	Converses stringing two to three sentences together; talks to others; expresses feelings; speaks about 200 words	Follows two- to three-step instructions; copies adults and friends; shows concern for others' feelings; understands 900 words
By four years	Knows basic grammar rules; sings or says poems; sings from memory; tells stories; knows first and last name; uses 2,200-word vocabulary	Differentiates real from make-believe; understands *same* and *different*; points to colors and knows what's missing; completes activities; matches and sorts; understands 2,500–2,800 words
By seven years	Plans oral presentations; reads grade-level books aloud; describes poetry components; uses vocabulary appropriately; aware of others' speech mistakes	Maintains eye contact; uses gestures; summarizes main points; analyzes readings; writes for different purposes;[2] understands 20,000–26,000 words[3]

1. U.S. Department of Health and Human Services, Centers for Disease Control and Prevention, "Learn the Signs: Act Early," pp. 1–2, www.cdc.gov/actearly (accessed March 28, 2013) and American Speech-Language-Hearing Association, "How Does Your Child Hear and Talk? Speech, Language, and Hearing Developmental Milestones," asha.org/public/speech/development/chart.htm (accessed March 28, 2013).

2. American Speech-Language-Hearing Association, "Your Child's Communication Development: Kindergarten through Fifth Grade," www.asha.org/public/speech/development/communicationdevelopment.htm (accessed March 28, 2013).

3. Comeunity, "Speech and Language: Causes, Milestones and Suggestions," www.comeunity.com/disabilityspeechguildelines.htm (accessed May 7, 2013).

and starts, flying through one developmental marker but pausing every so often, seemingly to gather strength, before moving on to the next plateau or stage of development.

Along the way, individuals develop their own way of talking and at their own pace. Think of differences in how friends speak. One may talk quickly, with words spilling out like a fast-flowing waterfall. Another may speak so slowly you want to finish every sentence for the person. Others may speak softly, loudly, or with a high- or low-pitched tone. They may hesitate before finishing a sentence, like President Obama, or insert "um" or "ah" between phrases. Or they may choose difficult words or very long sentences to express themselves, while others respond with few words simply put. These speech and language differences fall within typical ranges of development. When any difference becomes too extreme and extends outside an acceptable range, a speech and language problem can occur.

Producing Speech

Human speech involves many body organs working together in a complex fashion. The entire process takes exact timing and nerve and muscle control. The brain sends messages to and from the lungs, mouth, nose, ears, and their controlling muscles. All these parts enable speech production in addition to breathing and eating. Quite complicated processes!

The vocal tract provides the source for speech production. Picture a single tube running from vocal folds in the larynx to the lips (see figure 1.1). A side branch extends to the nasal cavity, or nose. Vocal folds in the larynx contain

It's in the Genes

Recent research revealed a language gene, technically called FOXP2 in science speak. Scientists first discovered this gene's capabilities to influence language after observing the same gene in chimpanzees and humans. They noticed that the gene switched on or off a network of other genes, especially in the brain, which is the control center for communication. The result was a theory that FOXP2 directly or indirectly causes chimps to communicate by grunting and humans to speak words. Research into the meaning of these results is ongoing. But the hope is to someday identify specific genetic causes for different speech and language disorders, such as stuttering, attention-deficit/hyperactivity disorder, and autism, so targeted treatment can be created.[c]

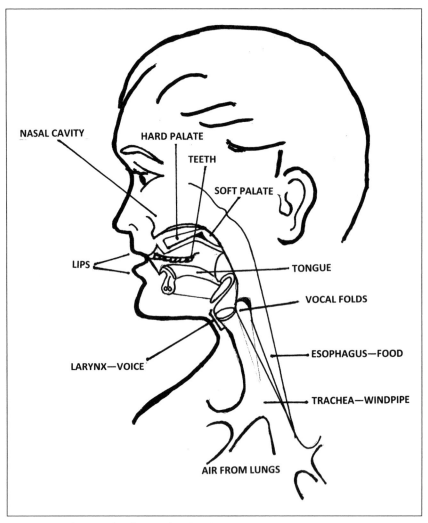

Anatomy of speech. *Illustration by Anne Ryan.*

muscles that are controlled by speech centers in the brain. Speech sounds arise from air exhaled through the trachea from the lungs and forced through the vocal tract. The way the vocal cord in the tract opens, closes, and vibrates contributes to how teens produce a range of speech sounds.

The upper end of the vocal tract, or oral cavity, contains the tongue, pharynx, hard and soft palates, lips, and jaw. These movable parts are important to speech production because the size and shape of the lips, tongue, palates—even teeth—can be altered. The slightest adjustments vary how sounds are produced. For example, when someone produces sounds in the upper regions of speech production without use of the lungs and back of the throat, they sound like Donald Duck. But someone who has lost front teeth produces totally different sounds. The space where the teeth had been causes a new way of moving the tongue, which disrupts regular flow of sounds. A problem in any area—brain, vocal tract, lungs—can disrupt speech.

When It's Time to Get Help

Teens want to express themselves in ways they choose. And they want to be understood by others. This may not always be possible. Problems communicating can appear suddenly or develop over a long time. Difficulties may be lingering and unresolved from early childhood. In addition, speech and language difficulties may appear together, compounding the problems, or separately. Whatever the situation, most speech and language problems can be improved. If anyone finds that communication isn't happening on a consistent basis, it's time to seek professional assistance. But where does someone begin?

A family doctor is a good place to start. Depending upon the issue, a doctor may recommend seeing an audiologist. Audiologists specialize in preventing, diagnosing, and identifying hearing loss not connected to another medical condition or treatment. Audiologists test ears together and separately in a sound-proof room with specialized equipment that transmits signals about what is heard. Readings from the equipment alert ear doctors to different types of hearing loss, which ears are involved, whether the hearing problem can be reversed, and whether hearing loss is affecting communication.

Once hearing loss is evaluated or ruled out, doctors usually refer communication problems to a speech and language pathologist (SLP). These therapists help people improve the ability to convey meaningful messages through language, the main goal of communication. SLPs are trained to evaluate how someone speaks. They want to identify if the person has a problem and what it is. Treatment sessions that follow incorporate activities designed to reduce speech, language (written, reading, and when English is a second language), swallowing, voice, and other specific issues. Therapists also work to improve what they call *social pragmatics*. This area involves social aspects of getting along better at home, school, and work with a communication disorder.

Where to Go For Help

If the family doctor cannot suggest a referral for an audiologist or speech and language pathologist, consult the American Speech-Language-Hearing Association (ASHA). Besides great information online or by phone and state-by-state referrals, the association certifies professionals. The group makes sure someone has the education and practice to become a speech and language pathologist or audiologist. So it is a good source to check before starting any therapy to ensure your professional is knowledgeable. Check the ASHA website, www.asha.org/about/contacts, to locate names of certified therapists near you.

"We have a mixed practice of clients ages two to ninety. I work with older kids transitioning to adults and preteens and teens as a classroom collaborator. The rest of the educational community recognizes that speech and language pathways play a big role in reading and writing. We give a lot of academic support to clients."
—Joanne Hein, Hein Speech-Language Pathology, Inc.[d]

Individual sessions at school might provide classroom support. For students with specific learning disabilities that involve language, therapy includes assistance with reading and writing. Students learn skills to organize class projects and express themselves to complete the projects. For students with autism or who use English as a second language (or English language learners, depending upon where someone lives), focus may be on expanding vocabulary and identifying which situations warrant using certain phrases and sayings. Other students may work on activities to help them feel more comfortable expressing themselves.

Initial sessions involve a speech therapist watching and hearing how a teen speaks. The therapist might record the teen saying particular sounds and words to determine how they flow. Teens may imitate sounds in front of a mirror or play games that build speech and language skills. In addition to activities during speech sessions, students may get exercises to practice at home. Just like improving in sports or with musical instruments, the key to making headway in therapy is practice.

SLPs may work for a public or private school district, so assistance becomes part of the regular school day. Or pathologists work at a public or private clinic, hospital, rehabilitation center, government agency, or college, or independently in private practice. Teens in therapy see pathologists one-on-one or in group sessions, depending on their individual needs.

Know Your Rights

Speech, language, and hearing therapy sessions can be expensive. Many teens have been involved in therapy since early childhood, which means lots of sessions and potentially big bucks. Usually, families of school-age offspring are not responsible for payments. If the need for a speech pathologist results from brain injury from an accident, insurance often allows for a given number of sessions. For teens in school, it's the law.

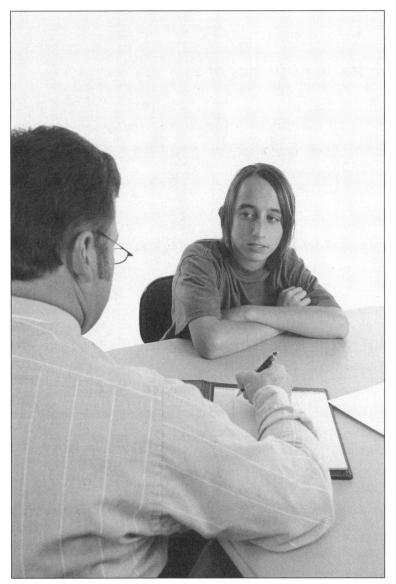

Speech therapists take a family and communication history as part of the evaluation process.

Under the federal Individuals with Disabilities Education Act, or IDEA, students qualify for paid in-school assistance, if a student meets the following definition: "(11) Speech or language impairment means a communication disorder, such as stuttering, impaired articulation, a language impairment, or a voice impairment, that adversely affects a child's educational performance."[1]

This means that once a qualified school pathologist tests a student and establishes a need for speech and language services, the school is required to provide those services. The school adviser, homeroom teacher, or special education educator or therapist will work with teens and their parents to devise an education

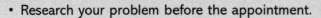

Planning for an Audiology or SLP Visit

Whether this is a first audiology or speech and language visit or a return to therapy with a new pathologist, consider these suggestions to make the most of the sessions.

- Research your problem before the appointment.
- Call ahead of time if you need an interpreter.
- Plan ahead what to ask the therapist.
- Write the questions on paper or your computer, so you won't forget anything.
- Keep a list of medications you may take, including supplements, handy. Some affect speech and hearing.
- Bring extra paper and pen or a laptop to write down what you learn in the session and information about exercises you need to practice at home.
- Discuss your main problem and the goals of the session(s).
- Ask how what you do in sessions will have an impact on your daily activities.
- Bring another person to help you remember what was said. Discuss the session afterward to make sure you heard everything correctly.
- Ask questions about anything you don't understand.
- Contact the therapist if there is anything you don't understand, even after the session. Ask the therapist the best way to communicate: e-mail, phone, meeting, Skype.[e]

plan that fits the individual student's needs. The written document, called an Individualized Education Program (IEP), sets goals to reach in therapy that school year. The IEP even designates a means of reviewing these goals on a regular basis. The IEP allows for other considerations to aid communication, such as electronic devices or extended time for tests. "We do lessons and therapy keyed into those IEP goals," said Keri Gold, licensed speech pathologist in Lake Zurich, Illinois.[2]

Depending upon the school district and IEP guidelines, schools offer a range of situations to enhance learning. Some schools offer classes that are cotaught. With coteaching, one teacher handles the academic subject for all students in the class, while the other is a special education teacher. The special education teacher is mainly responsible for adapting regular class material as needed and making sure that students get the accommodations listed in their IEPs. Special educators provide the repetition and building of one task upon another that helps support individual students during and after class.[3]

Another high school learning option is called supported education. In this situation, an aide stays in the classroom with an individual to answer specific questions, reteach material, and provide accommodations, such as reading tests aloud to the student or allowing extra time with assignments, that are spelled out in individual IEPs.

Not all speech disorders require extra assistance in the classroom. Some teens go to resource classes. These are a version of special education study hall. A special education teacher or speech pathologist who understands study strategies helps kids plan and use time better. Students who take advantage of this support, usually do better in class. The speech therapist works with teachers, parents, and other professionals involved in following the student's individual guidelines to improve communication skills.

Resources

Organizations

American Speech-Language-Hearing Association
2200 Research Boulevard
Rockville, MD 20850-3289
301-296-5700
nsslha@asha.org
A professional association for 150,000 audiologists, SPLs, and speech, language, and hearing scientists that offers professional accreditation, general communication information, advocacy, the latest research, and access to therapists.

Brain Injury Association of America
1608 Spring Hill Road, Suite 110
Vienna, VA 22182
703-761-0750
www.biausa.org

Advocacy and general information about dealing with problems arising from traumatic brain injury.

Family Resources Center of Disabilities
11 East Adams, Suite 1002
Chicago, IL 60603
312-939-3513
www.frcd.org
Information and referral services about special education rights.

WHEN WORDS WON'T FLOW: STUTTERING AND OTHER FLUENCY CHALLENGES

When normal fluency occurs, the rate and continuity of speech production flow at a regular pace. Most people develop these patterns of speaking when they're very young. Even babies babble and jargon in free-flowing patterns. Once they add sounds, syllables, and words and sentences, these, too, take on particular verbal fluency.

Susannah's Story: In Her Own Words

I entered private speech therapy when I was four years old because I had difficulty articulating certain sounds. When I was five years old, I began to stutter. At this point the focus of my speech therapy switched to stuttering because it had become more of an issue. I went to speech therapy for seven years. When I was eleven, I participated in a three-week intensive stuttering program at a local college with five other kids and teens who stuttered. We practiced techniques to reduce our physical tensions, and we dealt with our thoughts, fears, and avoidance behaviors surrounding stuttering. This was the first time that I met other children and teenagers who stuttered, and it was the first time that I really talked openly about my own stuttering.

I think my stuttering affected how I thought of myself more than how others thought of me. Stuttering was never a problem with my friends, and I was never bullied. It also was not a problem in school: I never allowed my stuttering to prevent me from participating in class or other high school activities. But I faced some negative reactions to my stuttering. I think most of these came from the listener feeling confused or uncomfortable.

After my freshman year of college, I returned to the college stuttering program for a refresher course with other adults who stutter. We again practiced strategies to reduce our physical tension and activities to face the psychological aspects of stuttering.

I was frustrated with myself at the end of this program because I had trouble maintaining the fluency. At age nineteen, I had entered the program thinking I had a healthy mental attitude about my speech and had already faced my fears of stuttering. I was wrong. I thought that fluency was successful and that if I diligently followed the steps outlined by this program, I would reach my goals. But working closely with the Stuttering Foundation as an intern, I was exposed to many stuttering resources as well as the larger stuttering community. I read books published by the Stuttering Foundation, and I listened to podcasts hosted by people who stutter (StutterTalk). Surrounding myself with these resources allowed me to realize that my journey with stuttering was far from over and needed to be on my own terms.

Now I'm twenty-two years old, and I recently graduated from college. I am currently working as a clinical research coordinator in the psychiatry department of a hospital. I no longer believe that I need to be fluent in order to be successful. I now strive toward reducing my struggle, and success means effective communication.[a]

Sometimes during early development, say, ages three to five, preschoolers might repeat or interrupt their flow of words. These are usually not permanent. Probably most teens can remember a time when they were so excited as a child— or perhaps more recently—that they said repeatedly, "Daddy, Daddy, Daddy?" or uttered something like, "C-c-c-ome quick! L-l-l-look at this!" They were so surprised they gasped before being able to say the first or last word in the sen-

"I had a scary experience in about eighth grade. For some reason, a neighbor told my mom I might have a speech problem, possibly stuttering. My parents started hanging on every word I said. Talking at home stressed me out because I thought everyone was watching and waiting for me to mess up. Pretty soon, I felt myself having trouble speaking. I had difficulty being fluent. I got even quieter than I normally was. Kids at school called me "Mumbles." But deep down, I knew I didn't have a speech problem, just a lack of confidence. Once I stopped reacting to what others thought of me, my speaking improved."[b]—Marlee

tence. Although others may mistake such instances as a fluency problem, these temporary patterns usually never turn into an ongoing issue.

When disruption in the natural, smooth flow of speech continues, as Susannah experienced at a young age, teens may have difficulty with fluency, also called *disfluency*. In most cases, disfluency begins in early childhood. Fluency problems that develop in teens or adults usually result from brain trauma, extreme illness, or severe emotional crisis. Discounting these, the two main fluency disorders teens experience are stuttering and cluttering.

Stuttering

Who Stutters?

Stuttering is the most common fluency disorder. Those who stutter account for about 5 percent of all children in the United States. That's more than 3 million individuals. Since one in twenty people stutter, chances are, if you don't stutter, you will encounter someone who does in your lifetime.

Part of the reason for this frequency is stuttering doesn't discriminate. The disorder affects families from all income levels and all walks of life. Stuttering can be found in any country, and people can stutter in any language. In fact, teens who stutter in their birth country and move to the United States, stutter in their new language, too. Worldwide about 68 million people, or 1 percent of the population, stutter.[1]

Like other forms of disfluency, most stuttering first appears during preschool years. As mentioned, though, a few cases begin later in life. Up until age four, both girls and boys stutter at an equal rate. For some reason, in children whose stuttering persists beyond four years, boys stutter more than girls. About four males stutter for every female.

No one is sure why generally boys seem to exhibit more problems—including other speech disorders, learning disabilities, and behavior issues—than girls. Some research has found differences in how boys and girls acquire language. Other studies discuss differences in how each gender is treated at home or school—or a combination of the two forces. While these assumptions are interesting, they do not totally account for the gender differences. And they really have little bearing on the fact that someone is left to handle the fluency problem.

Receiving early therapy reduces the number of stutterers dramatically. Three-quarters of children who participate in therapy for their stuttering when they're young find they no longer stutter by late childhood. That leaves only about 1 percent with a problem lasting into high school and adulthood.[2]

Although leaving class for therapy might not suit everyone, speech therapist Suzi Shulman found that her students relished their time together. "Students who stutter need to feel comfortable in situations where they can talk freely. They like speech therapy because they feel most comfortable with their therapist. They think, 'I can stutter in front of her and won't be judged.' A safe place for them to go is important."[3]

Dancing to Fluency

Twenty-year-old Shane Garcia made it to the Las Vegas round of season ten (May 2013) of television's *So You Think You Can Dance* but got cut from the top twenty. Still Shane, who stutters, is a star to many people who fear stuttering in public. Judge and actress Minnie Driver noted, "When people have to say something, they find a way to say that."[c] Shane's communication tool was dance.

"Being that I stuttered over the years, I've found different methods to mask it. When I make a beat [with his hands or feet] and talk to the beat, I can talk more fluently. I use dance as my language."[d]

To Shane, these tryouts on television proved more than his talent. They proved that he can do anything, despite stuttering. During tryouts, Shane communicated through his bone-breaking and Haitian movements. "I want to inspire at least one person not to let anything hold you back. I'm through with that."[e]

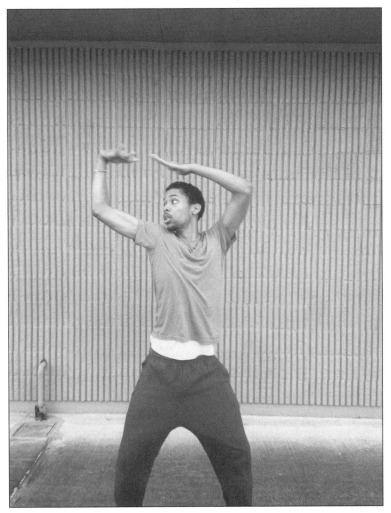

Shane Garcia, age twenty, communicates through his bone-breaking form of dancing. *Courtesy of Shane Garcia.*

What Is Stuttering Like?

A common sign for teens who stutter is the inability to utter sounds or words when they choose to speak. Beyond that symptom, stuttering takes on different characteristics with each person. To describe different ways someone may stutter, speech pathologists use four key terms: blocking, bouncing, prolongation, and repetition.

Imagine opening your mouth to speak and words not coming out. Therapists call this *blocking*. It happens when air from the lungs gets stuck in the vocal folds rather than being released through the throat and mouth. When silent blocking occurs, speaking is almost impossible.

As the speaker struggles to talk, frustration builds. That's when tension builds, and you might see physical signs of someone trying to speak. The face turns red and contorts from working hard to get words out. Veins bulge. Eyes blink. The body jerks or shoulders tense. One man who stutters held up his hands, like jazz hands, when he got stuck trying to say the word *hand* or the *h* sound. Any or all of these physical signs signal the stress of trying to talk.

Once air flow begins again, a burst of words might erupt. This seems as if the speaker is trying to rush every word out before blocking starts again. Some stutterers make inhaling, exhaling, or different sounds instead.

In other instances, those who stutter may repeat sounds and syllables quickly, such as, "f, f, f, f, f." They sound like they can't move on to a different sound. Another term for this pattern of speaking is *bouncing* because the sound seems to skip, or bounce, as it is repeated rapid-fire.

Some speakers who stutter prolong certain sounds, like a sneeze that won't come out, "a——choo." They may linger on the sound for longer than necessary for regular speech, for example, "m————oney." Therapists call this speaking pattern *prolongation*. Still others who stutter may repeat the same syllable several times before being able to move onto another syllable or word, such as "Whe-Whe-Whe-Whe- Where are you g-g-g-g-going?" This speech pattern is called *repetition*.

Stuttering emerges in different patterns. One person may stumble on certain sounds. Another may have difficulty starting sentences or new thoughts. A few teens stutter in addition to other speech and learning problems. Stuttering can be mild, moderate, or severe, depending on how frequent and regular interruptions are. Some people interrupt every sentence they utter, while others can speak with an occasional stutter on specific sounds.

What Causes Stuttering?

Historically, theories of why people stutter have focused on psychological or character disorders. Superstitious early cultures believed that people who stuttered were just evil. So tongues were burned to wipe out "black bile." Or the wagging part was boiled in wine to unfreeze what wasn't working right.[4]

Some early or superstitious cultures believed preferring the left hand over the right indicated evil intent or shame in the person involved. By the nineteenth century, doctors figured the problem was the shape of the tongue, so they surgically altered it by removing wedge shapes. But all surgery did was leave a lump that produced poorly articulated sounds.[5]

Theories that pegged personality as the cause for stuttering persisted into the twentieth century. Many professionals thought those who stuttered suffered from mental disorders. They were a nervous lot. They talked too fast or were overly

The Lazaro Effect

Tryouts for the 2013 season of *American Idol*, the popular television talent show, turned into some of the most emotional in the program's history. That's because one of the contestants stuttered—and badly. Twenty-one-year-old Cuban American Lazaro Arbos worked hard to answer questions and explain himself to the judges. But almost every sentence proved a struggle. His mouth twisted. His eyes blinked and opened wide. His hands waved, as he tried to express himself when words stuck in his throat.

The judges listened patiently but looked doubtful Lazaro would be a good prospect for the show. Lazaro noticed their looks, but he forced himself to stay positive. His dream was to sing on stage, which he had never done. This was his big chance.

Lazaro began singing, "Bridge over Troubled Water," a song that expressed his journey with stuttering. To everyone's amazement, his stuttering disappeared. He sang in a clear and beautiful voice. More importantly, the words flowed naturally: no halting bursts of words that infected every sentence he uttered earlier. When Lazaro finished, people in the audience bolted from their chairs and erupted in applause. Judges agreed with their enthusiasm for this singer. They sent Lazaro to the semifinals, then the final top ten.

"Ever since I was small, I wanted to sing," Lazaro told a reporter. "You can't let yourself get down."[f]

Lazaro developed a significant stutter by his sixth birthday. At the time, his family lived in Cuba. His teacher yelled at him to "talk right," but that never helped.[g] When his family immigrated to Naples, Florida, he was ten. The move only worsened his stuttering. Lazaro learned English quickly. Now he stuttered in English and Spanish—and on almost every sentence.

"No one wanted to hang out with me at class. I had no friends, so I stayed home," Lazaro said.[h]

Lazaro received speech and language therapy throughout school. By age thirteen, his therapist still counted him stuttering thirty times in two minutes, a huge problem. That year Lazaro received a hearing aid–like electronic device that creates background noise. Some stutterers find the background sounds mask their disfluency, so they stutter less. The device helped, but Lazaro continued to stutter. The only time he didn't stutter was when he sang. Sometimes his mother would tell him to sing what he wanted to say.

Lazaro graduated from high school in 2009. Without much confidence and few friends, he took a job scooping Italian ices. He figured it was the "only job I can get where I don't have to do 'smart people' stuff like talking."[i]

Still he kept alive his dream of singing. When tryouts for the twelfth season of *American Idol* were announced, Lazaro headed for Chicago. He wound up lasting through the season until he was the last male standing. Only five other contestants, all females, remained on the stage—an amazing feat, especially for someone who stuttered.

"Six months ago I never rode a plane by myself, I never did anything by myself," Lazaro said after being eliminated from *American Idol*. "I want to meet my fans so bad. I love to travel, so I'd love to see the whole country."[j] Lazaro showed that people who stutter can dream big and succeed.

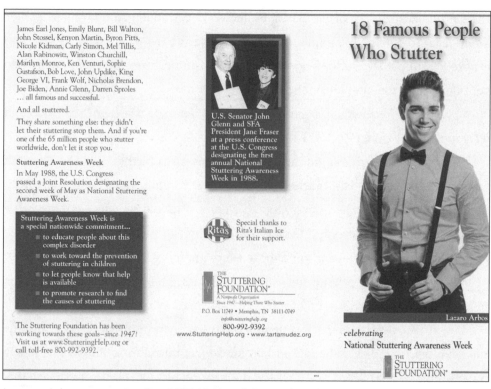

Lazaro Arbos on poster for 2013 National Stuttering Awareness Week. *Courtesy of the Stuttering Foundation.*

Lazaro's brave singing in public inspired others who stuttered to take chances, too. In Australia, eighteen-year-old Melvin Victoria watched as Lazaro sang week after week on the show. He saw how Lazaro thrilled audiences enough to keep voting him back.

Melvin had never heard someone who stuttered like he did on stage. Watching Lazaro inspired him to try out for his country's *Idol*. With a voice so sweet that it brought tears to listeners' eyes, Melvin wowed the judges. Melvin finally allowed himself to dream of one day singing professionally like Lazaro. A reporter called Melvin's success the "Lazaro Effect."[k]

shy. They fidgeted. Or they had bad parents, who corrected their speech until they stuttered or caused severe emotional or physical trauma that led to stuttering. More recently, times—and thankfully better-researched theories—have changed these assumptions. New technology and scientific advances have made controlled study possible.

Many stutterers feel that if they can discover what causes their particular stuttering, they can cure the disfluency. That's easier said than done. The exact cause of stuttering is still unknown, although many believe the nervous system plays a key role. Scientists are moving closer to finding precisely how stuttering originates.

Research points to several causes, some working in combination. Recent studies focus on stuttering as something that runs in families. Between 50 and 70 percent of people who stutter have a family member who either stutters or has another communication problem. In fact, children with an immediate family member who stutters are three times more likely to stutter themselves. The reason is in their DNA, or genes. Several studies have located nine different chromosomes involved in stuttering, reinforcing the family connection. *Chromosomes* are the tiny strands in genes that carry traits inherited from one or both parents, such as eye and hair color or how tall someone becomes.

Not every family member who carries stuttering genes will stutter, but certain families encounter clusters of members who do. For some young children who have a family history of stuttering, the condition may be triggered by having trouble responding verbally on command, being "unable to meet verbal demands." The combination of extreme stress and genetic makeup that leans toward stuttering seals their speaking fate. To date, however, no single common gene has been found to cause stuttering, so genetic research continues.[6]

Stuttering in the Movies

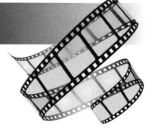

Media has not always depicted stuttering—and those who stutter—in a positive light. The few characters who stuttered in movies presented severely flawed personalities. The more common stereotype assumed those who stuttered were either extremely shy, overly nervous, or totally tortured human beings.

Actors who stammered (another word for a form of stuttering) appeared as violent criminals in *Taking of Pelham 1-2-3* (2009) and *Primal Fear* (1996). One actor played an abused and suicidal patient in *One Flew Over the Cuckoo's Nest* (1975).

The 2010 addition to stuttering in movieland involved actor Colin Firth as England's King George VI in *The King's Speech*. George VI was the unprepared royal who suddenly rose to the English throne when his brother gave up that right. Firth depicted a likeable enough person. But his stuttering was blamed on emotional problems that are considered myths today.

The storyline recalled his overbearing parents who refused to let him write with his left hand, even though he was clearly left-handed. As a young child he wore a painful metal brace to straighten his knock-kneed legs. He had an abusive nanny. All these could be difficult experiences for any young child. But they are not causes of stuttering.

The king suffered many therapy trials throughout his life. The movie opens with him trying to talk with marbles in his mouth to avert a stutter. He was told to smoke in the misguided attempt to control breathing patterns and stop his stuttering. Neither treatment worked.

Then an Australian speech therapist, Lionel Logue, played by Geoffrey Rush, swooped in to help the nervous king lessen his stuttering. Logue was well-known for his novel methods of improving public speaking. He guided the king through breathing and relaxation exercises. He had the king talk while wearing headphones that blared music. He made him sing, dance, and curse to get out words, all distracting—and revolutionary—ideas at the time. Logue told the king to prepare for speeches by practicing tongue-twisters. In the end, the king still stuttered. But he now felt comfortable enough to talk to the public on radio and in front of crowds.[1]

"It's all over my family, and a lot of us stuttered as children but got therapy early on," said Jane Fraser, daughter of the Stuttering Foundation of America founder, who also stutters. "None of my generation or their children or their grandchildren have that problem."[7]

For some teens, birth-related head trauma—such as trauma caused by the use of forceps or by stroke or brain injury—play a role in their stuttering. A difficult birth may cause cerebral palsy or mental retardation, both conditions that may disrupt the ability to coordinate muscles and nerves involved in speaking fluently.

Recent studies also link stuttering to brain differences. The Stuttering Foundation reports that brains of those who have stuttered since childhood differ from those with fluent speech. Regular speech usually originates from the left side of the brain. But brain scans of those who stutter show that the right side takes over tasks handled by the left, which scientists call *rewiring*. A defect in the brain's motor cortex shows on the left, the part that controls movement. This defect disrupts instructions to throat and mouth muscles.

A researcher from the University of Goettingen in Germany found evidence that those who stutter have difficulty relating what they say to what they hear. He described the resulting disfluency as "music from a disorganized orchestra. The question is not single elements themselves, not the instruments. They all know their parts. The question is how to activate them in a coordinated and well-timed fashion," researcher and neurologist Martin Sommer said.[8]

Evidence of brain involvement comes from other studies that found some people who stutter have more trouble with understanding and decoding auditory cues than their nonstuttering peers. Those who stuttered scored higher on language development. But they had greater difficulty hearing differences between sounds and words and reproducing them correctly. The defects in how stutterers process sounds causes a delay in responding. That contributes to uneven speech.[9] Some parents described their child's problem as the "mouth can't keep up with his brain."[10] These difficulties are linked to the brain, too, specifically the cortex.

Stuttering Does Not Affect Language

Many people work around their stuttering by finding a profession that doesn't involve speaking. Writing is a prime example. Check out these famous authors who stuttered but still had a way with words: Lewis Carroll (1832–1898), Margaret Drabble (1939–), Francine du Plessix Gray (1930–), Henry James (1843–1916), Edward Hoagland (1932–), Philip Larkin (1922–1985), Somerset Maugham (1874–1965), and John Updike (1932–2009).

Another theory being investigated proposes that stuttering results from fluctuations in *dopamine*, a chemical in the brain that affects motor control over speaking. According to this theory, the body of those who stutter produces too much dopamine. Increased dopamine levels usually occur as a natural response to stress. Certain individuals, like those who stutter, might be oversensitive to the chemical. As a result, smooth speech suffers from the slightest increase in dopamine.

Researchers struggle to determine the importance of social and biological factors in causing stuttering. How much does a troubled upbringing, overbearing parents, or bullying influence stuttering? Certainly, any of these situations can make someone anxious and worsen stuttering. But they are not causes. Sorting through reasons why someone stutters allows therapists to target a specific treatment.

Through the years, several myths have become popular about what causes stuttering. Here are some of the most common ones that are simply untrue:

- *Poor fluency is the stutterer's fault.* Nothing could be further from the truth. Whether research targets the nervous system or brain chemicals or anything else, the list of possible causes does not blame the person who stutters.
- *Stuttering is catching, or contagious.* Someone cannot catch stuttering by being near someone who stutters, like a cold or by hearing him or her stutter. As mentioned, stuttering comes from something inside teens who stutter. Either they inherit the genes that may cause disfluency, or they have problems with development of their nervous or motor systems.
- *Stuttering comes from stress.* Old theories focused on stress as a cause of stuttering. Certainly stress and anxiety may make fluency more difficult. But these factors cannot make someone stutter who is not already prone to the problem.
- *Stuttering results from the same reasons someone has lower intelligence.* As with other speech challenges, listeners often assume someone who stutters is not very bright. This is another way-off-base assumption. Studies show that people who stutter have the same range of intelligence, enter the same range of professions, and go to college at the same rate as those who never stutter. No connection exists between intelligence and stuttering.
- *People who stutter can control their disfluency.* This is a classic case of blaming the person with the problem. Stuttering is inborn and varies with different conditions. Treatments don't always work for given individuals. Appropriate treatments may take a long time to find, if at all, and last for years. Finding the right treatment takes lots of time and money. If teens could control their stuttering, they would know the cause and how to "cure" it, which cannot happen.

How Is Stuttering Discovered?

Stuttering may seem obvious to anyone who hears someone stutter. But an exact diagnosis by a trained professional is necessary before treatment can begin. A speech and language pathologist looks at a combination of factors before making a determination. First, a complete case history is taken. Therapists want new clients to explain when they first noticed speech differences and when stuttering occurs more frequently. They ask whether there is a family history of stuttering or any other speech, language, and learning problems. They want to know if someone ever had therapy and, if so, what kind.

After taking a history of stuttering—by talking or answering written questions—pathologists want a speech sample of how the teen talks. They analyze speech and language abilities and stuttering behaviors they might hear. How often does stuttering happen? What type of breaks in speech are heard? How does the teen respond when fluency lags? The therapist evaluates how long stuttering has continued, family history, probable causes, and severity of the stutter and other problems to create a complete picture. Then the therapist predicts whether the client will outgrow stuttering and what type of treatment might work best and for how long.

What Are Treatment Options?

Early cures seem comical today. They ranged from nutmeg under the tongue to holding someone's feet while they talked. Then there was the recommendation to hit the child's mouth with a dishrag. Needless to say, none of these odd treatments worked. Nowadays therapists realize that no complete cure for stuttering

> "I was born with an interestingly different brain, and as a consequence, I had many emotional problems growing up. I stuttered. I had phobias and tics and all sorts of anxious habits. . . . My stuttering was the most tormenting problem though. . . . I remember once sitting at the dinner table and literally being unable to speak the words, 'Pass the butter.' So my mother said, 'Sing it.' And even though it was embarrassing to break into song in front of my family, I did just that, completing the sentence in one try. That single incident momentarily lifted a tremendous burden from my shoulders, proved to me that, if worse came to worst and I couldn't speak, I could always sing."
> —Carly Simon, songwriter, singer, stutterer[m]

exists. Therapy sessions can go on for years, often with questionable lasting effect, or end in childhood. The work to reduce disfluency can be slow and difficult. At times, stuttering may seem completely gone, only to reappear at a later time.

That said, several helpful treatments are available. But the type of treatment that works for one person may not work for another. Choosing different options depends on age and what someone wants to accomplish from treatment. One teen may need coaching for a job or college interview. Another may want to feel more comfortable on a date or speaking in class. Many more hope to reduce stuttering overall. Talking with the speech therapist is the best way to begin identifying communication goals and the range of treatment alternatives.

Most therapists apply a multipronged approach to treatment. Up-front discussions between therapist and the person who stutters help dissect any emotional issues associated with troubled speaking patterns. Which speaking situations contribute to stuttering? What attitudes or emotions does someone harbor about his or her stuttering that would interfere with progress and increase disfluency? Sessions with a trained counselor, psychologist, or speech pathologist can help with adjustment and attitude issues.

Speech and Language Therapy Sessions

Current therapies for kids and teens aim to find ways to lessen stuttering. Sessions help people understand their stuttering, what contributes to disfluency, and which words and situations cause greater fear. Once teens objectively understand what they are dealing with, they can begin to reduce fears of speaking.

More important, teens can bolster their self-image and take charge of how they act—and react—when stuttering occurs. Often, just deciding to actively participate in something constructive to diminish stuttering can be a confidence builder. Working on both disfluency and reducing sensitivity to what others think about stuttering can be empowering.

Therapists may recommend teens audiotape or videotape themselves while talking. They can hear how they sound, which may not be as bad as they think. And they can objectively hear and see improvement, as they participate in therapy.

Another key aspect of enhancing fluency is learning to change stuttering patterns. Exercises to improve breath control and speaking patterns aid stuttering management. Stutterers learn to:

- focus on speaking more slowly and deliberately.
- prolong vowel sounds, rather than certain consonants. Voiced consonants cause more stuttering than voiceless. Examples of voiced consonants include *b, d, g, m, n, w, r,* and *y,* while voiceless consonants are *p, t, k, f, h,* and *s.*

- relieve muscle tension by positioning the tongue and lips in a way that eases sound production.
- feel movement of vocal cords as they produce sounds.
- hesitate between words, sentences, and thoughts to adjust air flow.

Sessions generally progress from practicing the smooth flow of single syllables to words to complex sentences. As with developing any skill—from learning an instrument to playing soccer—practice increases chances of improvement.

Teachers and parents may be included in the therapy plan as a way to help teens who stutter. Coordinated efforts provide support and continuity. As teens age, though, they are not necessarily interested in another round of therapy *or* talking about therapy, communication problems, or anything else with more adults. But they may harbor any number of feelings—frustration, embarrassment, anger, fear—about a speech problem that won't go away. Therapists and other adults in their lives are there to help, not create more problems.

Drug Therapy

Although a magic drug to eliminate stuttering sounds great, no approved drugs to treat disfluency exist. Some doctors prescribe drugs that alleviate related conditions, such as anxiety or depression, for stuttering. But these medications are mostly ineffective for disfluency. Even if they alleviate the problem temporarily, a bigger problem with these drugs results from the side effects they create. Uncomfortable and sometimes strong reactions make these medicines difficult to take for very long. The National Institute on Deafness and Other Communication Disorders is funding research to investigate other forms of drug therapy.[11]

Electronic Devices

Some people who stutter find electronic devices helpful with controlling fluency. The devices fit into the ear like a hearing aid and create an echo or masking sound. The idea of exposure to background noise to ease stuttering is based on observations that many people stuttered less when they spoke as part of a group. For unknown reasons, the echo fooled the brain into thinking others were talking. Moreover, those who stuttered could not hear their own voice as easily. This masking of one's voice allowed the speaker to relax and talk more fluently. But improvement lasts only a short time. This is what Lazaro Arbos, the *American Idol* contestant who stuttered, discovered. Researchers continue to examine these and other devices for their long-term effectiveness.

Self-Help/Support Groups

When problems, any problems, become overwhelming, talking to others often helps. No one knows what stuttering involves except another person who stutters. That's why doctors and therapists often recommend a support group for teens who stutter.

The combination of speech therapy and self-help, as in a group setting, proves the most successful for many people with disfluency. Remember to consider online chat rooms, especially if being anonymous suits your personality better or you feel less self-conscious speaking in a group that cannot see or hear you. Several sources for groups with people the same age are mentioned in this chapter's Resources section.

Teletherapy

Enter the modern age. Some therapists offer therapy sessions remotely via computer. They supply the same activities but at any hour that's convenient for therapist and client. The best part is therapy happens in the comfort of your home. The therapist learns more about your home environment, and you get to practice being more high tech while saving time and money without a commute. Teletherapy gives stutterers in remote areas a way to receive the same quality therapy as someone near a medical center or in a large city.[12]

Wild and Crazy Reactions to Stuttering

Let's face it: stuttering makes some listeners uncomfortable. They fidget. They look away when you talk. They look for excuses to escape. Some listeners feel so impatient that they finish your sentences. Or they tell you to slow down, thinking these words will magically make disfluency disappear. Or they want you to "think

Singing without Stuttering

Seems strange, but many people who stutter when they speak, sometimes severely, never stutter when they sing. That's the case with popular stuttering songsters Carly Simon, B. B. King, Nancy Wilson, and Mel Tillis. How is this possible?

Scientists offer several reasons for this remarkable ability. One has to do with the brain and how differently it processes talking and singing. Spoken language uses the left side of the brain, while singing requires messages from the right side. So singing eliminates processing words through the side that has difficulty making them flow.

Another explanation focuses on how vocal cords, tongue, and lips form words differently with singing than with speaking. Singing allows words to be prolonged, which reduces chances for stumbling. And singing is a smoother process in general that is easier on the voice. No pressure. Controllable time factors. That's why speech therapists suggest singing to practice emitting words fluently.

In fact, some people who stutter benefit from any change in speaking that allows them to focus more on presentation than the words. Many find stuttering relief by whispering, speaking to a rhythmic beat, or expressing themselves in a higher or lower pitch than usual. Acting provides another way to shift speaking patterns. Perhaps the ability to assume another persona besides that of a stutterer allows someone with a disfluency to never stutter on stage.°

about what you're saying," as if you aren't already focusing on how difficult it is to talk with them.

But these reactions are their problems, not yours. For anyone who stutters, it's important to realize that you are going to encounter the same ups and downs as other kids. These experiences rarely have anything to do with stuttering. Think about interacting with the opposite gender, which can be scary. What about worry over an important test, something every student experiences? What about interfering parents: what parent isn't? All these are separate issues from stuttering—and all situations every maturing adolescent faces. Boosting self-confidence to handle whatever happens can go a long way toward dealing with reactions to stuttering from others.

Decide to Make Progress

Sadly, stuttering sometimes seems overwhelming, even with everyday interactions. You respond to others' reactions by not speaking at all, such as never answering the phone at home. You avoid situations where you need to speak, such as going to parties or places where classmates hang out, or you only say words you know will flow naturally. Your parents may complain that you are rude because you refuse to answer the phone or door or participate in family conversations. Those who stutter are not alone, as most teens have felt similarly at one time or another.

If you decide to participate in your treatment, success will usually follow. Hiding and fighting involvement or pretending you don't stutter takes energy. This is energy that would be better applied to productive therapy sessions and other aspects of your life. Above everything else, as one adult said looking back on growing up, "Don't ever give up!"[13]

Dealing with Parents

One of the most helpful suggestions from those who stutter is to be honest with those close to you. Parents may not want to bring up stuttering, or you may not want them to know how difficult your stuttering has become. Both sides may worry they have somehow failed or disappointed the other. So the topic hangs in the background like the proverbial elephant in the room. Instead, parents may let you get away with more than siblings because they feel terrible or guilty about the stuttering. Or they may do embarrassing things, like talk for you or finish your sentences, in an effort to be helpful.

They—and friends, teachers, and classmates who react similarly—won't know how offended you are unless you tell them. Being honest is the best thing you can do for yourself and those around you.

> "Because of my stuttering, I quit school after completion of eighth grade and remained out of school for three years. . . . I did not use the telephone until I was seventeen, and my parents did my shopping for me."
> —Dorvan Breitenfeldt, former professor at Eastern Washington University[p]

Lil JaXe: Rapper, Stutterer

Sometimes teens have to be creative when disfluency makes life difficult. Jake Zeldin knew about disfluency because he stuttered all his life. When he was ten, he discovered that when he rapped his stutter disappeared. Now he writes sentences and rhymes that he performs without a hitch, even when on a television talent show or with reporters. The rapper calls himself Lil JaXe. His rapping gives him another way to present school assignments and communicate with friends—and a cool way at that![q]

Ask for regular scheduled talking time at home. Make sure family meetings occur when no other activity conflicts to remove time pressures of conversing. Write your concerns, if you feel you can express yourself better that way. Don't hibernate because you stutter. Your family wants to help you.

Taking Stuttering to School

The same hints apply for teachers at school. Most teachers have little experience with stuttering. They may harbor misconceptions about your intelligence because you hate to read aloud, do not answer questions, or seem unusually shy with classmates. School personnel may be uncomfortable when a student stumbles when speaking. Most teachers want to help ease your time in class. You need to help them.

The only way for teachers to know how to help, however, is if you give them input about stuttering. You have to advocate for yourself and take the initiative.

- Talk with teachers about stuttering either before entering a new class as an introduction or once classes have begun. Schedule a meeting when the teacher isn't overloaded. You want to avoid time pressures, which can increase stuttering. Take the lead in assisting teachers with dealing with their feelings about stuttering. Explain that if they and classmates stay calm and unemotional when you speak, fluency will come easier. If a meeting isn't possible, write a letter of introduction or explanation.
- Suggest ways to include someone who stutters in class activities that involve speaking. Offer that more time with answering is one way to increase comfort with responding aloud. Request advance warning, if possible, for reading in class, so you can practice beforehand.

- Emphasize that people who stutter want to be treated like everyone else. Special treatment is just as isolating as not talking. If teachers want to help, suggest that they ask you, the school therapist, or your parent(s) for ideas as well. Request that information about a student who stutters be part of a substitute's lesson plans, so the substitute is not surprised and wanting to interrupt you during class activities.
- Remind the teacher that finishing sentences or telling someone to calm down or hurry up only creates more disfluency.
- Develop together ways to handle classmates who laugh or bully because you stutter. Maybe the teacher can remind classmates that everyone has problems with something. In your case, the issue is with speaking naturally. Or you could devise statements ahead of time that diffuse the discomfort someone who teases may feel about your stuttering. For example, you could make an offhand statement about your trouble speaking, such as "I have difficulty saying this sound. I'm working to say it better," or "That didn't come out right, did it? Better luck next time," or "I'm not nervous: I just stutter and need more time to talk than you do."
- Prepare a class presentation about stuttering. Most bullying and jokes comes from fear and ignorance. Arming classmates with solid information about stuttering will reduce their discomfort about someone who stutters. Perhaps you could promote National Stuttering Awareness Week, the second week in May, as a way to educate classmates. Since 1988, different groups in the United States have used this time to build awareness about stuttering. Check out other helpful hints for reducing stress in certain situations in chapter 9.

Cluttering

Another fluency disorder similar to stuttering is *cluttering*. Some therapists call cluttering the orphan of fluency problems because little has been written about it. Since fewer people encounter cluttering, stuttering gets all the attention.[14] Partly this information lag is due to how relatively new the disorder is. Although some therapists have mentioned cluttering symptoms for decades, researcher Desco Weiss first published one of the earliest explorations of cluttering during the 1960s. Since then, authors have rarely addressed issues of cluttering. Mainly speech and language professionals and those who experience the disorder are familiar with the term. As a result, cluttering is often misdiagnosed or not considered at all. But with more than half of those who stutter also having a cluttering problem, the disorder deserves more attention.

The primary characteristic of cluttering is speech delivery that either races, is irregular, or is a mixture of both. Speech can be slurred to the point of being

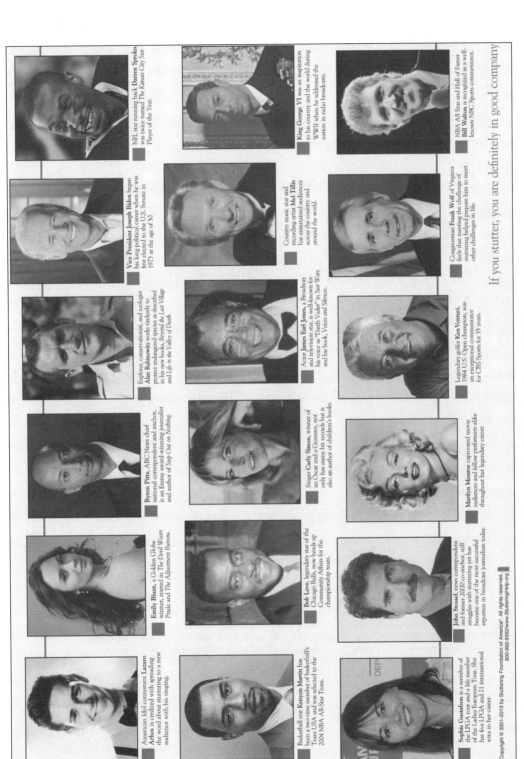

NFL star running back **Darren Sproles** was twice named The Kansas City Star Player of the Year.

King George VI was an inspiration to his country and the world during WWII when he addressed the nation in radio broadcasts.

NBA All Star and Hall of Famer **Bill Walton** is recognized as a well-known NBC Sports commentator.

Vice President **Joseph Biden** began his long political career when he was first elected to the U.S. Senate in 1973 at the age of 30.

Country music star and recording artist **Mel Tillis** has entertained audiences across the country and around the world.

Congressman **Frank Wolf** of Virginia feels that meeting the challenge of stuttering helped prepare him to meet other challenges in life.

Explorer, conservationist, and zoologist **Alan Rabinowitz** works tirelessly to protect endangered species as described in his new books, *Beyond the Last Village* and *Life in the Valley of Death*.

Actor **James Earl Jones**, a Broadway and television star, is well-known for his voice as "Darth Vader" in *Star Wars* and his book, *Voices and Silences*.

Legendary golfer **Ken Venturi**, 1964 U.S. Open champion, was an exceptional commentator for CBS Sports for 35 years.

Byron Pitts, ABC News chief national correspondent and anchor, is an Emmy award-winning journalist and author of *Step Out on Nothing*.

Singer **Carly Simon**, winner of an Oscar and a Grammy, not only has many hit records but is also an author of children's books.

Marilyn Monroe captivated movie audiences and fellow performers alike throughout her legendary career.

American Idol contestant **Lazaro Arbos** is credited with spreading the word about stuttering to a new audience with his singing.

Emily Blunt, a Golden Globe winner, starred in *The Devil Wears Prada* and *The Adjustment Bureau*.

Bob Love, legendary star of the Chicago Bulls, now heads up Community Affairs for the championship team.

John Stossel, news correspondent and former 20/20 co-anchor, still struggles with stuttering yet has become one of the most successful reporters in broadcast journalism today.

Basketball star **Kenyon Martin** has been a two-time member of basketball's Team USA and was selected to the 2004 NBA All-Star Team.

Sophie Gustafson is a member of the LPGA tour and a life member of the Ladies European Tour. She has five LPGA and 21 international wins in her career.

If you stutter, you are definitely in good company

Eighteen famous people who stutter. *Courtesy of the Stuttering Foundation*

unintelligible. The difference between disfluency in stuttering and cluttering is speakers who stutter know what they want to say but can't express the words, while with cluttering, words sound disorganized, as if the speaker is unsure of what to say. When speaking, clutterers sound confused and can't seem to retrieve the right words. Often cluttering overlaps with other learning and speech disorders, such as stuttering, attention-deficit/hyperactivity disorder, learning disabilities, and other auditory procession problems. A similar range of mild to severe symptoms exists with cluttering as well as stuttering.

Cool Folks Who Stutter

Teens may hear that stuttering isn't cool. Or that those who stutter are not as smart in class or don't have friends. Or they'll never amount to much in life because of how they talk. Well, listen up. People who stutter achieve the same range of successes—and failures—as anyone in the nonstuttering population. And they have the same range of skills and talents and goals to use them well. This list shows that people who stuttered learned to live with stuttering and become standouts in their fields.[r]

Marc Anthony, pop singer, two-time Grammy winner, and three-time Latin Grammy winner

Joseph Biden, vice president and career politician who first was elected to the U.S. Senate in 1973 at age thirty

Emily Blunt, actress

Wayne Brady, television host and comic

Steve Brill, creator of *Court TV*, a magazine, and an airport security company

Johnny Damon, Tampa Bay Rays outfielder and top major leaguer in runs, hits, and stolen bases

Sidney Gottlieb, psychiatrist and chemist

Sophie Gustafson, five-time Ladies Professional Golf Association winner and top golfer in twenty-one international tournaments

Bo Jackson, multisport professional athlete

Samuel L. Jackson, actor

James Earl Jones, actor in theater, television, and movies who is known for his rich voice, including as Darth Vader in *Star Wars*

Nicole Kidman, award-winning actress

B. B. King, legendary blues guitarist, singer, and songwriter

John Melendez, comedian, actor, and musician

Alan Rabinowitz, zoologist, conservationist, and author

Shaquille O'Neal, former NBA star and current television sport's analyst

Budd Schulberg, Oscar-winning screenwriter and noted novelist

Carly Simon, singer and songwriter

Mel Tillis, country music singer and songwriter who received honors from the Country Music Hall of Fame and Grand Ole Opry

Diagnosis

Speech and language pathologists evaluate cluttering in much the same way as stuttering. The difference is a more extensive questioning that includes information about other learning and behavior problems in school or at home. Therapists require longer, more involved screening samples to distinguish cluttering from other problems and evaluate differences between someone's slowest and faster speaking rates.

Treatment

Therapy for cluttering depends upon what else might be involved. The American Speech-Language-Hearing Association recommends several procedures for treating cluttering, some similar to those for stuttering. They involve:

- using creative techniques to help someone who clutters talk slower. Slowing the rate of speech allows extra time to organize and express thoughts.
- helping teens who clutter monitor their own speech.
- reinforcing good sentence structure that is coherent. Therapy begins with short simple sentences that become more complex as cluttering lessens. Clutterers learn to describe what they say after it is said, so they learn to organize messages.

- listening exercises, so someone who clutters learns the normal give-and-take of conversation. Listening also provides positive role models for sentence structure and speaking.
- reducing profound disfluencies through activities similar to those used with stuttering. In fact, since some cluttering is masked by stuttering, activities to lessen stuttering are given first. Only after stuttering is removed as an obstacle can therapy tackle cluttering.[15]

Resources

Organizations

Friends (the National Association of Young People Who Stutter)
38 South Oyster Bay Road
Syosset, NY 11791
866-866-8335
www.friendswhostutter.org
National organization for young people who stutter and their families that holds annual and regional conferences, produces a bimonthly newsletter, and runs mentoring and graduate student training programs for those who want to pursue careers in treating stuttering.

National Stuttering Association
119 West 40th Street, 14th Floor
New York, NY 10018
800-WeStutter (800-937-8888)
www.westutter.org
Organization that offers support and information to the stuttering community, organizes conferences, and prepares quarterly newsletters.

Our Time Stutter
330 West 42nd Street
New York, NY 10036
212-414-9696
www.ourtimestutter.org
Nonprofit organization started by stuttering actor and director Taro Alexander that uses the arts to boost confidence and communication skills for kids and teens who stutter. The group offers therapy, summer camp, newsletters, and mentoring and other programs in the New York area.

Speak Easy International Foundation
233 Concord Drive

Paramus, NJ 07652
www.speakeasyinternational.com
International support group for all-age people who stutter.

Stuttering Forum
www.stutteringforum.com
Free website for posting and participating in stuttering-related discussions, linking to products/therapies, and connecting with others who share the joys and concerns of living with stuttering.

The Stuttering Foundation of America
P.O. Box 11749
Memphis, TN 38111-0749
800-992-9392
www.stutteringhelp.org
Nonprofit organization dedicated to providing information/brochures about prevention and treatment of stuttering and a nationwide referral list of specialists who treat stuttering. The organization website has a section for parents, another for kids, and another for teachers, each with tips for fluency and articulation disorders.

Books: Nonfiction

Apel, Melanie Ann. *Coping with Stuttering*. New York: Rosen Publishing, 2000.
  Description of stuttering, causes, and treatment.
Curlee, Richard, et al. *Do You Stutter: A Guide for Teens*. 4th ed. Memphis, TN:
  The Stuttering Foundation, 2004. Defines stuttering and issues teens who
  stutter may experience.
Logue, Mark. *The King's Speech: How One Man Saved the British Monarchy*.
  New York: Sterling, 2010. Condensed timeline of how an Australian therapist
  helped ease the stuttering of King George VI. The story is based on the therapist's diaries and was the basis of a movie of the same title.

Books: Fiction

Frank, Lucy. *Lucky Stars*. New York: Atheneum, 2005. Thirteen-year-old Kira
  hates that her father makes her sing on subway platforms, but classmate Jake
  longs to vocalize anything without stuttering.
Fusco, Kimberly Newton. *Tending to Grace*. New York: Alfred A. Knopf, 2004.
  A compelling story about a teen who happens to stutter and is forced to make
  her own way when her mother dumps her at a quirky aunt's farm.

Olswanger, Anna. *Greenhorn*. New York: New South Books, 2012. A small (forty-eight pages) book that pacts a huge punch. The middle-grade+ story centers on a young Holocaust survivor and how he protects a little box he carries with him everywhere. For his secretive protection of the box and the fact that he stutters, the Jewish school student suffers terrible taunts. Eventually, he finds a friend—and his voice—and the horrific mystery of the box is revealed.

Shields, David. *Dead Languages*. New York: Alfred A. Knopf, 1989. An ironic, sometimes funny yet painful, coming-of-age story about a teen with a terrible stutter whose parents both make their living with words as writers.

Vawter, Vince. *Paperboy*. New York: Delacorte, 2013. Award-winning novel about the difficult encounters an eleven-year-old boy who stutters experiences after he takes over his friend's paper route.

DVD

Kaplaglu, Semish. *Bal (Honey)*. United States: Olive Films, 2011. Yusuf, an only child living with his parents in the isolated mountains of Turkey, finds the strong bond with his beekeeper father cannot protect him from being shunned in school because he stutters. Yusuf grows silent when his father must travel on risky business.

MIXED-UP SOUNDS AND WORDS: SPEECH SOUND DISORDERS

Young kids often say versions of sounds and words that many consider adorable. Toddlers and preschoolers mix up letters and say funny things like "nana" for "banana." Or they replace one letter with another, such as saying "das" for "gas." These speech differences usually fall within a normal developmental range. Sometimes, however, cute speech turns into habits that persist long past the age when they are considered normal. Not so cute anymore!

In such cases, parents need to suspect a speech sound disorder. Teens with a speech sound disorder have significant difficulty communicating sounds that are appropriate for their age. Usually, the errors make speech difficult to understand. This is especially true for strangers who are unfamiliar with the speaker.

Have you ever met someone whose parents or best bud explained an entire story that didn't jive with what you heard from that same person? Or talked with an older relative or someone who was in an accident—one that might have produced a stroke or other brain trauma—who now distorts sounds enough to make understanding that person difficult? These situations may be the result of the speaker exhibiting a speech sound disorder that, if not corrected, interferes with communication. Whenever you believe your speech is causing worry or embarrassment, no matter at what age, you need to seek help.

The number of people with a speech sound disorder varies with age. Usually, these issues get addressed during early grades. Thereafter, the number of students with speech sound disorders drops from 24.6 percent before age five to about 1.06 percent by junior high and high school. But problems can continue into adulthood if not eliminated or reduced through therapy. As with stuttering and other speech disorders, males get a raw deal. They display greater impairment more frequently than females. Rates of at-risk females to males range from 1.5 to 2.4.[1]

Don't Let Trouble Talking Silence You

Sometimes, having a speech problem feels like a kick in the confidence gut. You stop talking in public. You blush, get nervous, or sweat when speaking to others. Inside, you may feel your heart race or get queasy at the mere thought of speaking. Speaking in front of a group is totally out.

To counter these feelings, you need to take better care of yourself. That begins with building confidence. Knowing on the inside what you can do successfully will help you project a can-do attitude on the outside. So find something you like to do, whether a subject in school or extra-curricular activity. Make sure the activity is something that makes you happy. Music, sports, volunteer jobs—all these can help you meet new friends and build confidence from your success. Discover other helpful suggestions at the website ShyKids.com.[a]

Defining Speech Sound Disorders

The American Speech-Language-Hearing Association (ASHA) divides speech sound disorders into two main categories: *articulation* and *phonological processes.* Articulation refers to how specific sounds are made. Are specific sounds left out, added, replaced, or distorted? Phonological processes refer to a pattern of saying the wrong sounds, such as substituting a single sound for words that begin with two consonants, for example, "soken" for "spoken" or "bing" for "bring."

A primary example of an articulation speech sound error is a lisp. With lisping, a teen usually substitutes the letters *s* and *z* with the sounds for *th.* In another example, someone might add sounds to words, such as saying "pinanio" for "piano."

People with articulation problems or phonemic disorders are as smart and aware as anyone else. With articulation challenges, teens know which sounds they cannot pronounce. But teens with a phonemic disorder, although aware of other aspects of their life, fail to differentiate certain sounds from the ones they produce. For example, someone might hear the word "cap" but say something closer to "tap." They might hear the distinction clearly but not be able to distinguish enough to repeat the correct word.

M's Story

Speech-language pathologist Caroline Bowen hosts a website where teens and young adults can share feelings about lisping. M wrote that he had a lisp since he started talking. Now he's fourteen, and his problems speaking continue, although he's had some therapy. He can't explain how bothered he is about his speech. The comments he overhears. The making fun of him at school and everywhere he goes. Kids can be so cruel. Even M's closest friends tease him about how he talks, often behind his back. When he has to speak in front of the class, he actually sweats when his turn comes. Usually, M tries to stay silent, so he won't get teased. "Everyone thinks it doesn't bother me, but it really does," he wrote. M's dream is to join drama club, but he can't because of how he speaks.[b]

Phonemic disorders go beyond saying the wrong sounds. In some instances, such as with the cap/tap example, the meaning of the word changes as well as the sound. Saying the wrong word, even when you never mean it, can be embarrassing in school, social situations, or any place else. Others may think you are not as smart because of what comes out of your mouth, which is untrue. Or listeners might not get what you request, which can be problematic at the store or in class.

According to ASHA, 80 percent of people with phonological disorders find them severe enough to require professional treatment. Moreover, between 50 and 70 percent of students experience difficulty with academic subjects, such as reading, math, writing, and spelling, in addition to their speech problem. So it's important to investigate and continue with speech and language support in school, even when you grow tired of the extra sessions and being singled out for therapy. Academic success may depend upon the extra support you receive.

What Causes a Speech Sound Disorder?

Isolating the specific cause of a speech sound disorder can be difficult. Some people with the disorder never learn why their problem exists. For maturing young children, an articulation disorder may stem from never learning correct methods of saying letter sounds or words. The children may place parts of their mouth in the wrong position when producing sounds. If not corrected, placement becomes ingrained and continues into upper grades. One study predicts that preschoolers

Regular Folks Who Mispronounce Words in Public

As with any speech problem, many folks gained fame in spite of their trouble talking. Sometimes this fame came from careers that require speaking in public. Check out these successful people from a variety of fields who have had a speech sound disorder—and become successful.

Humphrey Bogart, famous actor who had a lisp

Rudolph Giuliani, former New York mayor who mispronounced sounds

Elton John, singer, songwriter with a lisp

Anthony Kiedis, singer (Red Hot Chili Peppers) with a lisp

Anybody Killa, rapper with a lisp

Michael Phelps, swimmer with a lisp

David Sedaris, author and comedian with articulation challenges

Mike Tyson, boxer-turned-author/actor with a lisp

Barbara Walters, television journalist who has difficulty pronouncing her r's. This articulation problem was so obvious that Gilda Radner, an original *Saturday Night Live* comic, became known for her character called Baba Wa-Wa, who highlighted Walters's speech sound disorder

And what list would be complete without the well-known characters with speech sound disorders who populate our cartoons: Donald Duck, Daffy Duck, Sylvester the Cat, Elmer Fudd, and Tweety Bird. They remind everyone to accept and laugh about differences.

with speech error patterns will likely distort sounds until they reach grade school and find they have an ongoing speech sound production problem.[2]

For example, a lisp sound results from placing the tip of the tongue between upper and lower teeth, instead of behind the teeth where it belongs for regular speech. This placement error produces an *s* sound common with a lisp. Frequently, listeners who don't understand speech sound disorders, or any speech and language disorder, believe that speakers with a speech sound disorder appear or are trying to sound younger and less knowledgeable than they are.

Lisping: A Gay Thing or Not

Too often, unthinking people who stereotype assume males who lisp are gay, whether they are or not. To test the assumption that all males who lisp are gay, linguistics professors Henry Rogers and Ron Smyth identified and recorded the speech of twenty-five men, seventeen of whom described themselves as gay. The researchers then asked several volunteers to listen to the recordings and identify which men they thought were gay or straight. The results indicated that listeners found identifying who was gay based on their speech difficult, as only 62 percent of listeners pinpointed the speakers accurately.

"Fewer than half of gay men sound gay," Rogers told *University of Toronto* magazine (June 2002). "The straightest-sounding voice in the study was in fact a gay man, and the sixth gayest-sounding voice was a straight man."[c]

The concept of lisping and gayness has many curious speech experts speculating on the stereotype. Some believe certain gay men adopt speech—and language and body movements—they think will help them adapt within the gay culture. Accommodation is much like how young children adapt to the language of their family. With speech and language, some—but not all by any means—gay men produce typically feminine behaviors that add to the stereotype. But lisping is not a gay problem: it can happen to anyone—male, female, gay, or straight.

"For some reason, I've been seeing more tongue thrusts in my practice," said Illinois speech and language pathologist Suzi Shulman. "Usually, these are corrected much earlier than junior high school or high school, but many students don't have access to therapy and can't afford private therapy or don't know they can be helped."[3]

In some cases, hearing loss interrupts normal speaking. Since communication is a blend of hearing and speaking (see chapter 1), teens who cannot hear correctly naturally have difficulty producing sounds. Frequent inner ear infections or nerve loss can impair articulation because sounds from others are either lost or muted. Children with hearing problems may not hear specific sounds at all, or these sounds may appear distorted. With inner ear nerve damage, teens can still hear vowels and low-frequency consonants when others speak. But they may lose hearing of high frequency sounds, such as p, t, s, and f.[4]

Physical problems beyond hearing loss can contribute to articulation disorders. Genetics plays a role in some families. Close relatives who have speech and language problems may influence other family members, exposing developing children to a speech sound disorder as well. In other situations, brain damage to part of the brain that controls and weakens muscles may affect how the tongue and respiratory system work during speech. Conditions such as Down syndrome, cerebral palsy, or accidental brain damage alter functioning of nerve centers that control oral muscles. Uncontrolled muscles interfere with producing understandable sounds.

Another physical problem that contributes to articulation challenges involves changes or defects with the shape of bones, teeth, and muscles. These may block normal speech sounds. A common birth defect is cleft palate and lip, which can play a role in both articulation and phonological disorders. Cleft palates, which are on the top, back part of the mouth, leave the roof of the mouth open and a space between the nasal cavity and mouth. When the cavity is inside the mouth, it is a cleft palate. More often, the cavity cuts a path through the upper lip as well, which is called a cleft lip. Usually, cleft palates and lips are closed shortly after

Conner's Story

Conner hated meeting new people. He couldn't say his name clearly. He couldn't explain himself so others could understand. For as long as he could remember, he suffered with this communication problem. His therapist called it apraxia, a strange name in itself. The name refers to a neurological, or brain, condition that interferes with motor control over speech. Parts of the brain that control muscles affecting speech are somehow damaged. Conner feels like he has a loose connection in his brain that won't allow him to control muscle movements for speech sounds.

Some kids with apraxia find their lips, tongue, and cheeks are so out of control that they have problems eating. Luckily, Conner's condition is milder, but he thinks he'll be in therapy f-o-r-e-v-e-r. He talks slower than other kids. Classmates accuse him of talking like a robot because he tries to be so careful with his words. And he often has trouble saying correct words. When he said "potty," other kids laughed. But he wasn't trying to say "potty," just "thirsty." Besides laughing, kids just say he talks funny and won't stay around long enough to become friends and learn he's really a smart and likeable guy.[d]

birth. If not, speaking clearly can be severely compromised. Even when surgery closes the opening, scar tissue can impede accurate articulation.

How Is a Speech Sound Disorder Discovered?

The best way to determine whether a speech sound disorder exists is to find a qualified speech and hearing pathologist to evaluate speech production. The evaluation probably includes a hearing test to find out whether a hearing problem is distorting understanding and speech sounds enough to alter production of intelligible sounds.

Therapists screen how oral and motor body parts work. They analyze how sounds are used to produce words and sentences. They check if and how teens understand and use language during normal conversation. Several inventories compare how developing adolescents articulate words with standardized norms. When all parts of the evaluation are considered, the therapist decides whether the person tested can benefit from therapy and, if so, what kind.

What Can Be Done for This Disorder?

The good news is habits begun in early years can be undone. Again, therapy sessions help. Articulation therapy from a trained speech and language pathologist

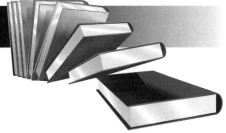

Good Read

A moving book that discusses an articulation problem is *Words in the Dust* by Trent Reedy.[e] The book is an amazing look at life in war-torn Afghanistan (beginning in 2001) and the brave girl who persevered in her dream of going to school. But she had three things blocking this dream. One was the war, and another was her family's belief that girls should marry and take care of children and the home. But she believed her greatest problem was her cleft palate and lip, a condition she had since birth. Neighbors taunted her because of how she looked. She feared going to the store or finishing chores outside the house. Then a group of American soldiers arranged for her to have surgery to repair her cleft palate. Afterward, her dream of an education was within her reach.

Roxanne Swentzell's Story: In Her Own Words

I do not know the scientific name for my particular speech impediment, but it was very hard for me to form words that were understandable. It would sound perfect in my head, but what others heard was just noise. I had this problem as soon as I could talk. I was sent to speech therapy throughout my elementary school years. The problem slowly corrected. I consider myself still learning how to talk.

Communication is vital to anyone. It was tremendously hard to not be able to tell someone something. I became very isolated at school and did not talk much. I stayed by myself a lot. I would get my sister to tell people things for me. I was made fun of in school, and it made me afraid to say anything. Not everyone teased me, so I did have some friends. I began to create a whole world in my art classes. I was not made fun of there but held up as a really good artist.

Because I struggled with language, I don't take speaking for granted. I think it has made me think more before I speak. I still work at forming words, and it can be tiring. I notice others not having this problem. My suggestion to anyone with similar difficulties is not to get so caught up in words. There is more than one way to communicate. Find another way to help you say what you are needing to say.

My speech problem helped me to become the artist that I am today. It forced me to learn a new language, the language of clay. And I believe this art form that I found to speak through relays more information than words can ever do. so I gained from my loss.[f]

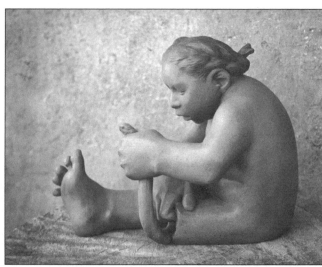

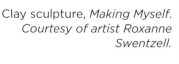

Clay sculpture, *Making Myself.*
Courtesy of artist Roxanne Swentzell.

Sculptor and Poet

Pueblo sculptor Roxanne Swentzell, who had her first one-woman art show the same year she graduated from high school, finds many ways to speak—from sculpting to poetry. Check out what art—and poetry—mean to her.

Poems to My Sculptures
You clay people
who dance through
my soul dance right on
through
me. . . .
I sculpt to
reach out to you.
Hoping to go
past the words
and thoughts
that bring
us to a shallow
world.
Hoping to catch
a moment
direct connection
between your
soul
and mine.
Then, for that second,
we will remember
what is important.
In remembering
there is Hope.[9]

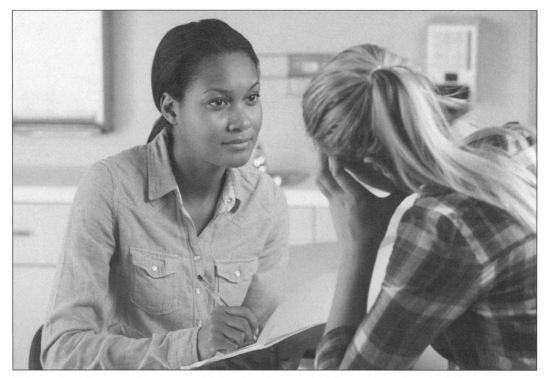

This student is arranging a cue with her teacher to alert her when misarticulation occurs.

targets articulation and phonological errors. The goal is to identify what is wrong, so the faulty sound or word choice can be corrected or modified. During therapy for articulation errors, teens might model what the therapist says. Or they may be trained to use visual and sound feedback, such as talking in front of a mirror. With phonologic disorders, teens may practice methods to organize what and how they will present to the therapist.

Once teens are able to identify when they misspeak, they can consciously work to correct the errors. In the beginning, adolescents may need assistance with awareness. The speech therapist may want to talk with teachers or parents to alert the teen about how the specific challenge sounds. Or teens can talk with a trusted teacher on their own. Teens can suggest a cue that alerts them to alter what was just said. Perhaps teachers can touch their ear to indicate a sound error. Or teens can arrange hand signs with a parent or older sibling. If teens in therapy misspeak, they see the gesture that alerts them to correct—or at least be cautious about future uses of that word or sound. The idea is to see a cue that warns but doesn't call unwanted attention to how someone speaks, which can be embarrassing.

"If articulation disorders last into middle school, many students are embarrassed and frustrated," Christy Cook, speech and language pathologist, said. "At this age level, they get teased more than other kids. They are less likely to speak

New Tools for Old Problems

Recent studies have reported that articulation problems can be corrected quicker with a set of tools called Speech Buddies. The set of five tools is designed by speech pathologists to correspond to five different articulation sounds. The five sounds covered are *r*, *l*, *s*, *sh*, and *ch*. By placing one of these tools inside the mouth, the device guides how the tongue moves when talking. Practice with the device allows the user to reinforce correct placement.

Testing shows after using the device the user is more likely to say the correct sound once the Speech Buddy is removed. Tests at various clinics and hospitals on clients of all ages resulted in quicker correct responses, cutting the usual twenty to thirty hours of treatment for an articulation disorder in half. Once a therapist shows correct placement of the device, the client can practice at home, which quickens results. Teens who used the devices reported feeling more confident as they were able to control how they talked.

Speech Buddies aren't cheap, however. In 2013, the complete set cost $299, and tools for individual sounds cost $149. But they may be available through school speech therapy or insurance coverage—and quicker response time to treatment brings down costs for individuals who are paying for their own therapy.[h]

in class, in front of others, or volunteer to read. Some adolescents are completely withdrawn. I have them record themselves to practice sounds, reading, and conversation. They have to practice—daily."[5]

Activities depend upon whether a specific cause was discovered during the evaluation process that needs to be addressed before sound production can proceed. Even if hearing is a problem that can be corrected, speech therapy is still needed to redo articulation patterns that existed when hearing was reduced.

Other activities the therapist may present include asking teens to respond to pictures, much like those from a Go Fish game. Students look for clues to differentiate sounds and practice repeating correct versions. Once they are successful at least 80 percent of the time, the therapist presents the next level of sounds to reproduce.

Speech Sound Disorders Go Way Back in History

Speech pathologists believe that famous Greek orator Demosthenes (born 384 BC), overcame an articulation, and possibly fluency, disorder. Demosthenes' speech had been difficult to understand since childhood. Yet, as an adult his speeches for law courts and on behalf of democracy were so highly regarded that he often was forced to present them himself.

Speaking in public became easier after an actor taught Demosthenes exercises to improve his diction. Thereafter, he became dogged about practicing. He created an underground hideout where he could repeat problematic sounds in private. While in training, he talked with pebbles in his mouth and recited verses while running along the water shouting over the crashing waves. To ensure he stayed hidden until he perfected the sounds, a process that often took two or three months, Demosthenes shaved one half of his head. He didn't want to be tempted to travel.

With time, his powerful speeches against government got him into trouble. He poisoned himself after government officials accused him of treason. But he went down in history as one of the greatest orators in Greek history.

A key plan for treating phonological disorders involves using pairs of words that differ by one sound. By presenting the two together, the therapist can focus attention on differentiating between the two sounds and definitions, if appropriate. Some therapists consider phonological problems as a language disorder, depending upon how someone sounds. In that case, treatment covers both the articulation and language aspects of communicating. The main goal of therapy for either speech sound disorder is to be able to use learned sounds alone and in blends outside therapy sessions in general conversation.

"I meet with parents and suggest they practice at home with their child. We speak all the time, and students should be aware of using teeth, lips, and mouth all the time to get muscle memory," suggests Cook. "I recommend that the teacher come up with nonverbal signals. If a student has trouble with *r*'s, for example, the teacher can make a signal to alert the student that the teacher is listening and will ask for a correction.

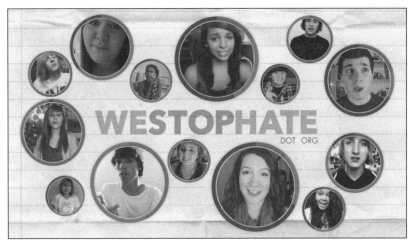

Teens participate in We Stop Hate, a program that promotes antibullying campaigns through its website, WeStopHate.org; YouTube videos; and Safe Space national in-school initiative. *Courtesy of We Stop Hate and founder Emily-Anne Rigal.*

Bullying and Teasing

Bullying is a problem for many teens. But it gets multiplied if you get teased—or worse—every time you open your mouth. You may hate to go to school. You may worry about responses each time you talk. The bullying may be verbal to your face, behind your back, or physical. Either way it hurts. You feel embarrassed, shunned, depressed, or anxious about your well-being. Schoolwork can suffer. You might become sick or lose sleep from the stress of being bullied. No way to live.

Time to take action. Here are some things you can do to rid yourself of the bully burden. Some of the following suggestions come from Matt's Hideout, a website created by a young adult from England who lives with dyspraxia and experienced his share of bullying in school.[i]

- Understand that you've done nothing wrong, and it's not your fault you are bullied. It's your right to attend classes and other neighborhood activities without the fear of intimidation.

- Keep cool. Bullies like when they upset the person they bully. It gives them power they may be lacking in the rest of their life.[j] Stay calm and walk away if you can. Or try a joke to diffuse the situation. Bullying can result in pent-up anger. Try to find an appropriate way of releasing the anger. And don't show the bully that he or she has gotten to you.
- Find friends to support you. Bullies like to get their prey alone. Find someone to walk with to class or home from school or activities. Join groups with like-minded people. Perhaps you can befriend someone else who gets bullied. There is safety and support in numbers.
- Stay near a person in authority or in safe areas of the school. Bullies are really cowards and won't approach you if they think they will get caught.
- Keep a diary of what is happening to you. A diary is a good way to get feelings out, but it's also a way to verify your experiences, should you need to show police, a school administrator, or a lawyer.
- Take care of yourself if you feel depressed. Talk with a professional, such as a counselor, doctor, or psychologist, if extreme sadness continues more than a couple weeks.
- Get help. You don't have to carry the burden yourself. Besides friends, talk with teachers, family members, or higher level administrators. Devise a plan with your teacher of how each of you should react when someone makes fun of how you talk. Teachers shouldn't allow any taunting in class against or from anyone. If the school isn't supportive, get your parents involved.
- Give a presentation about what your speech problem is and how it isn't your fault or something to make fun of or fear. Information often brings understanding.
- Organize others—kids and adults—to change the culture of accepting bullying. Request that your school prepare and distribute a clear outline about its bullying policy that protects all students, even those with speech problems. Write letters to local government officials about a community effort to get the word out that your community doesn't appreciate or accept bullies.
- *Never believe what bullies say about you.* You do not deserve their treatment. You are better than what they want you to believe.

"For parents, I say don't correct all day. I recommend dedicating a time, such as homework and reading aloud sessions, to practice speaking. Don't correct with regular conversation. The message is more important than how it comes out. Homework time is speech time."[6]

Resources

Organizations/Websites

Born This Way Foundation
bornthiswayfoundation.org
Organization started by singer Lady Gaga and her mother, Cynthia Germanotta, to encourage a safe society that is more accepting of individual differences. The group has a website and various activities and is supported by the Berkman Center at Harvard University and the MacArthur Foundation.

Cleft Palate Foundation
1504 East Franklin Street, Suite 102
Chapel Hill, NC 27514-2820
800-242-5338
www.cleftline.org
Nonprofit organization that provides information, research, and support to patients, families, and professionals about cleft palates and lips.

Kids Health
kidshealth.org/teens
Site devoted to a variety of topics related to growing healthy kids and teens, including bullying, homework organization, and public speaking anxiety.

National Bullying Prevention Center
Pacer Teens against Bullying
8161 Normandale Boulevard
Bloomington, MN 55437
800-537-2237
TTY 888-248-0822
www.pacer.org/bullying
Site for teens against bullying that offers resources, personal stories, and action plans to prevent and stop bullying.

ShyKids.com
www.shykids.com
Site divided into sections for different-age readers and parents that offers ideas and book suggestions about how to build confidence, overcome shyness, and make friends.

Southern Poverty Law Center
400 Washington Avenue
Montgomery, AL 36104
334-956-8200
www.splcenter.org
National advocacy and legal organization prominent in the battle to end discrimination and bullying. Its team produces amazing free classroom material (videos, *Teaching Tolerance* magazine, newsletters) and provides legal support when all else fails.

Speechville Express: Phonological Disorders/Teens
www.speechville.com/diagnosis-destinations/phonological-disorder/phonological-disorder.html/ and www.speechville.com/teens/older-children-talk.html
Site for teens, parents, teachers, and anyone interested in learning more about speech disorders, in this case, phonological disorders, insurance for therapy, where to locate a speech pathologist, and issues confronting teens, especially those with speech and language problems.

StopBullying.gov
www.stopbullying.gov
A federal government website managed by the U.S. Department of Health and Human Services that offers advice about bullies and how to stop them, research on bullying, and information about cyberbullying.

We Stop Hate
westophate.org
Nonprofit project started by teen Emily-Anne Rigal to stop the cycle of being bullied, then becoming a bully. The project has a strong web presence that is dedicated to building confidence and ending bullying. Lady Gaga and Meryl Streep are among celebrity supporters, as are several corporation sponsors.

WiseGeek
www.wisegeek.com
Site that answers questions about all types of speech and health topics.

Books: Nonfiction

Sedaris, David. *Me Talk Pretty Some Day*. New York: Little, Brown, 2000. Humorous memoir that has a chapter championing Sedaris's fifth-grade rebellion against speech therapy, which motivated him to learn a huge vocabulary and pursue a career with words.

Books: Fiction

Brill, Marlene Targ. *The Underground Railroad Adventure of Allen Jay: Antislavery Activist*. Minneapolis, MN: Lerner Publishing, 2012. Graphic novel historical fiction story about how eleven-year-old Allen, who had a cleft palate, made himself understood to a runaway slave, led the runaway to safety at the next Underground Railroad station, and grew up to become a well-known educator and lecturer.

Draper, Sharon. *Out of My Mind*. New York: Atheneum, 2012. Novel about a fifth grader with cerebral palsy who everyone thinks is dumb because she can't talk. Then she invents a technical device that allows her to speak for the first time.

WHEN THE VOICE GOES HAYWIRE: VOICE DISORDERS

At some juncture, everyone experiences voice problems. Most, like a raspy throat or low pitch, are short term and result from a cold or flu. These difficulties are definitely not extreme enough to be considered a disorder of any kind. But disturbances that stem from habits developed over time can harm the voice. When the voice is used in the wrong way, altered sounds result. Luckily, these habits can be corrected by voice therapy. Even when physical damage to vocal mechanisms contributes to voice changes, these too can usually be treated successfully.

How Do You Know You Have a Voice Disorder?

Usually, voice says a lot about how you feel. For example, when you are excited or angry, your voice may become louder than usual or strained. Ever listen to the comedian Lewis Black? He makes his points by yelling at the audience. Sometimes, he runs out of air before he finishes a sentence. Or he sounds hoarse toward the end of his presentation.

The key indicator of a voice disorder involves how you sound. If you constantly sound hoarse or raspy or breaking up, sound appearing and disappearing like a broken cell phone connection, you may have a problem with your voice. Another clue is when pitch suddenly changes, either rising high like a boy going through puberty or dropping low like an actor in a creepy movie. Or you may notice how often you run out of air before reaching the end of the sentence. Any of these manners of speaking that persist longer than two weeks may indicate a problem that could use professional help.

Sometimes others notice your voice problem before you admit to having one. Do people often tell you to talk louder or softer? Do you sound strange because

Melanie's Story

Melanie looked forward to starting her teaching career with fourth graders. After a few weeks of teaching, however, she found her voice so hoarse at the end of the day she couldn't speak at night. A few months later the problem became so bad she couldn't talk enough to teach. Her regular doctor referred her to an *otolaryngologist*, a doctor concerned with the ears, nose, and throat. This doctor discovered that Melanie had growths, one quite large, on her vocal folds. The growths, or polyps, inhibited the vocal folds' free movement, which prohibited sounds from flowing.

Since most growths on vocal folds result from using the voice improperly, the otolaryngologist referred Melanie for a voice evaluation by a trained speech pathologist. The evaluation showed that Melanie used the bottom range of her pitch when she talked while most people are supposed to produce a broader range of sounds. Melanie also spoke louder than necessary, not uncommon in the classroom. And she clenched her teeth, possibly from new-teacher tensions from trying to control unruly students.

After twelve weeks of therapy, Melanie's polyps almost disappeared. Once her vocal folds could move normally, her voice returned. Therapy helped her resume teaching, but she continued to apply the techniques her pathologist taught her. She monitored her pitch and loudness and made sure she opened her mouth wider when she talked. Opening the mouth wider resulted in a more relaxed way of speaking. And it preserved her career—and voice.[a]

you're too nasal, like too much air escaping from a hose, or not nasal enough because too little air is moving through the nose? Hearing constant complaints and concerns may indicate the need to see a doctor or speech pathologist for evaluation.

Speech pathologists take a case history and other voice measurements. They want to know what you think the problem is and how you feel about it. Therapists may want to observe you in different situations, such as at school and home, to identify possible voice abuses, such as yelling, and misuse, such as pitching the voice too high or too low. They will ask you to talk in a conversation and read a passage. As you use your voice, they complete rating scales that judge pitch, loudness, nasal quality, and rate of speaking.

> ## Discrimination and Voice Disorders
>
> What difference does having a voice disorder make? Turns out a lot. A recent University of Cincinnati, Ohio, study compared responses to a survey given to thirty-two teachers of female adolescents. The survey asked what teachers thought of students with normal voices versus those with a voice disorder. Results showed that teachers rated students with voice disorders lower than those with regular speech in a range of personality and academic traits. This led researchers to warn that "female students with voice disorders may be at risk for academic, social, and vocational difficulties." Study authors further suggested that people dealing with a voice disorder needed to be proactive on their own behalf. Investigators proposed educating those around them—teachers, classmates, friends—about what a voice disorder is and isn't. Remember: Knowledge is power—and builds understanding.[b]

Therapists assess physical structures involved in speaking, including facial muscles, teeth, hard and soft palates, tonsils, lips, and larynx. Sometimes, you will be asked to blow into a mouthpiece to evaluate lung air volume, airflow, and other aspects of breathing functions. A special device measures a recording of your voice for quality, such as the amount of vibrations or jitters.

Another device measures voice intensity, such as problems with loudness. This instrument also measures the intensity of how someone begins to speak. This is called *glottal attack*. Hard, abrupt eruptions can sound extreme, but they can also indicate speakers who come from large cities of the northeastern United States. In contrast, soft glottal attacks might suggest speakers from the rural southwest, but they can also reveal a problem when the attacks are extreme. All these tests contribute to deciding if you have enough of a difference speaking to require treatment for a voice disorder.

What Causes a Voice Disorder?

Voice disorders arise from a variety of sources. Anywhere air passes from the lungs, through the vocal cords, and on through the throat, nose, mouth, and lips can be the source of a defect affecting how someone sounds. Problems that contribute to voice disorders can begin after an illness or from other parts of the body. For example, continual acid backing up from the stomach during digestion can cause throat irritation that can result in vocal changes. A more serious condition, cancer of the throat, can alter tissues affecting the voice or contribute to growths on the vocal folds. Or a birth defect in the thin layer of tissue between vocal cords that evades early discovery can influence how the voice develops.

Some nasal speech arises from structural blockage in the nasal cavity that interferes with airflow. The cause can be allergies, a cold, or a growth. Once blockage goes away, so does poor nasal quality.

At times, overuse creates conditions that affect voice. Screaming, constant throat clearing, or continual singing stresses vocal cords and can result in voice

Vocal Paralysis Derails Songster

Born in 1990, singer, songwriter, and actor David Archuleta started winning singing competitions by age ten. After being named Junior Vocal Champion on television's *Star Search 2* at age twelve, he was sure singing would be his future. But by fourteen, David's doctor diagnosed him with vocal cord paralysis.

Vocal cord paralysis is a voice disorder that results when one or both vocal folds refuse to open and close properly. The kind David had, single—or partial—vocal cord paralysis, is more common and less life threatening, but it's still dangerous.[c]

The fourteen-year-old worried his musical career was over. He lost his range. He had trouble sustaining notes. "From the moment I got the diagnosis, life quickly went from *Star Search* to soul search," David said.[d]

Rather than give up, David worked with a speech therapist. He persisted in practicing the exercises the therapist recommended. With time, David gradually learned better breath control and was eventually able to speak without trouble. His singing improved enough that he became the youngest contestant in *American Idol*'s top ten (season seven).

He explained, "[I] still had a paralyzed vocal cord, but . . . my cords had found a way to work around the condition because by some miracle, they were vibrating despite what medically wasn't supposed to be able to happen. The one vocal cord, it seemed, had actually grown over and around the weak one in order to adjust for the other not working."[e]

Now David enjoys a budding career as an international singer and songwriter. He wrote about his experiences with vocal paralysis in a memoir titled *Cords of Strength: A Memoir of Soul, Song, and the Power of Perseverance* (2010).[f]

changes. If the problem persists without treatment for a long period of time, changes occur in tissues of the larynx. Over time, the changes can develop into nodules or polyps. These situations can contribute to the growth of noncancerous growths, such as cysts or ulcers, on vocal cords that interfere with the free flow of air needed for regular speaking.

Sound Like a Frog?

When someone is hoarse, what comes out sounds breathy, strained, and raspy. The throat might feel scratchy or raw. These are indicators of vocal fold problems.

Vocal folds are two bands of smooth muscle tissue that line the larynx. The larynx lies between the base of the tongue and the top of the trachea, or passageway to the lungs. When you are silent, vocal folds stay open, so air flows for breathing. But when you speak, the brain controls a series of events that trigger the vocal folds to vibrate as air from the lungs passes through them. These vibrations create sound waves that move through the throat, nose, and mouth.

Air flowing through these cavities determines how someone sounds. Voice, including pitch, volume, and tone, depends upon the size and shape of vocal folds and how they move air through the cavities. These differences explain why every person has a unique voice. Relaxed vocal folds create a deeper voice, while tensing them produces a higher pitch. For example, you can hear a speaker's tension in the rise of pitch when someone gets excited or angry.

Hoarseness can come from the similar range of conditions that create other voice disorders. A medical otolaryngologist can figure out the cause and what can be done to relieve the problem and prevent its return.

Laryngitis

Any cold, upper respiratory infection, exposure to harsh chemicals, or severe allergies can result in laryngitis. This condition is the most common cause of hoarseness. In extreme cases, laryngitis leads to gradual loss of voice and throat

Medical Alert

Warning: Never take decongestants to ease laryngitis. They can dry vocal cords, making matters worse. In addition, try not to whisper, as that strains the larynx even more.

discomfort. Depending upon the reason for laryngitis, a doctor prescribes rest, antibiotics for bacterial infections, or antihistamines for allergies.

Voice Misuse, Abuse, or Overuse

Not surprisingly, yelling, talking over friends at parties, screaming at a sibling, or cheering at sporting events can lead to laryngitis. So can excessive cell phone use or cradling a telephone handset on your shoulder. Teachers and lawyers often get hoarse from constant talking for long periods of time as part of their workday. So do singers, actors, and public speakers. In fact, you can hear presidential candidates slowly lose their voices as prolonged campaigns drag on. Problems develop when anyone speaks in public without proper amplification.

The strain of talking under difficult conditions abuses the vocal cords, causing inflammation and resulting hoarseness. So does talking loudly or using vocal cords inefficiently, straining them in unusual circumstances for lengthy time periods. Voice problems can result from excess tension in the neck and muscles of the larynx, such as from cradling a phone between the ear and shoulder. Poor breathing technique can also cause the voice to tire easily.

In addition, vocal abuse comes from the habit of constant throat clearing. When continually misusing the voice, thin layers of the vocal folds thicken. Think of what that kind of rubbing of vocal cords can do over the long term.

Other forms of misusing vocal cords result from a person's habit of smoking a couple packs of cigarettes a day. Smoke plus chemicals in the cigarettes dry the throat and who knows what else. Another form of vocal cord abuse is repeatedly

Bogart-Bacall Syndrome

Ever hear of the famous acting couple Humphrey Bogart and Lauren Bacall from the 1940s and 1950s? Besides being top actors and having a highly publicized marriage, the two shared recognizable sexy, husky voices. Bacall lowered hers on purpose to sound sexier in certain films. Bogart had a natural nasal twang, so he required special voice training, too. Both actors were so popular that anyone who developed vocal fatigue that strained the vocal cords was said to have Bogart-Bacall syndrome. The problem resulted from muscle tension in the larynx and neck. Tightening limited streams of air flow and caused an abnormally low-pitched speaking voice. Natural voice sounds can return with proper education and therapy.

Smokers Beware: Your Voice May Suffer

For thirteen weeks in 2013, singer and actress Bette Midler played chain-smoking agent Sue Mengers at a Broadway theater. The role required Midler to become a two-fisted smoker, smoking one cigarette after another. She often lit one cigarette while puffing down another. According to the storyline, one hand held a marijuana joint while the other fingered a regular cigarette. Midler, however, puffed on herbal cigarettes. Any smoking is too much when it comes to protecting the voice. Even in that short period of time, the result for Midler was a terribly strained voice.

"The cigarettes nearly killed me," Midler told a New York Times reporter. "I answer the phone now, and people think it's my husband. And my allergies in that very old theater. And the hair spray! But the cigarettes were the hardest."[9]

When it comes to protecting the voice, you don't have to be a famous actor or singer. In fact, several experts recommend not smoking and staying away from places that expose anyone to secondhand smoke. Smoking contributes to a host of ailments that can hurt the voice, such as acid reflux, changing how vocal cords operate, and cancer. Best to never start smoking—or work to quit.

---

ingesting over-the-counter decongestants for what is assumed to be nasal drip. That should be a doctor's call. Make it a habit to never take any medication unless it's approved by the doctor.

The best therapy for voice misuse is not using the voice at all, but that often seems impractical. Speech therapists offer vocal exercises and speaking tips that can help modify breathing and how the voice is used. There are also exercises to break a throat-clearing habit. For vocal abuse, stop smoking and stay away from decongestants. To prevent or ease hoarseness without therapy, drink at least six glasses of water a day, inhale steam, and apply warm compresses to the throat to relieve inflammation.

Gastroesophageal Reflux Disease (GERD) or Acid Reflux

Once thought a condition for older folks, GERD is becoming a problem for larger numbers of teens and younger adolescents. When you feel a burning sensation in the chest (also called heartburn) or stomach, discomfort in the throat (possibly like the stomach contents want out), or a sour taste in the mouth, those might

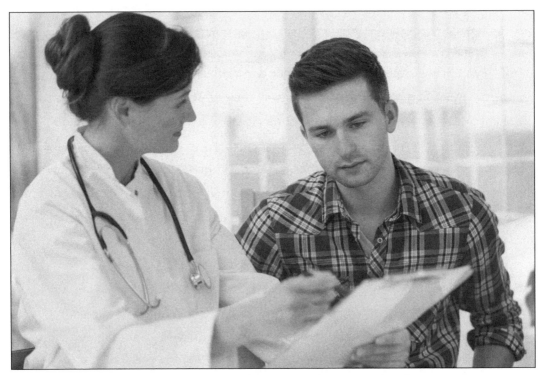

Check with a doctor to rule out GERD when acid backs up into the throat.

be signs of GERD. If you experience hoarseness, trouble swallowing, and a dry cough, these are other clues to head for the doctor. A doctor visit is in order, particularly if symptoms worsen after eating or lying down at night.

With GERD, stomach acid backs up into the throat. The backup irritates every internal organ along the way. Usually, food you eat goes through the esophagus and into the stomach. A muscle at the bottom of the esophagus shuts, so foods and liquids stay in the stomach. Inside the stomach, acids produced there digest, or break down, what is ingested. When the muscle either opens at the wrong time or cannot close properly, stomach acid moves backward (also called acid reflux) into the esophagus, causing the discomfort of GERD. Because this process happens automatically, you often do not know a problem exists until you experience persistent hoarseness or a troublesome cough or chest discomfort.

GERD is a medical problem. Therefore, anyone with these symptoms needs a physical exam from a doctor to determine if GERD is causing the hoarseness. Doctors may run tests to look for irritation. They may require special X-rays or a tube with a tiny camera threaded into the esophagus. These procedures may follow a spray to numb the throat or anesthesia to allow sleep, both designed to relax the patient.

In rare cases, symptoms result in a tear in the muscle that separates the abdomen from the chest, which would require surgery. Most often the cause comes down to what teens eat. Once a diagnosis of GERD is determined, the doctor will suggest lifestyle changes in what and how much you eat to ease the problem. If those don't work, your doctor may prescribe medication.

Why is GERD on the rise? Experts offer several reasons from smoking to drinking alcohol to weight gain. The reason mentioned for the increase most often involves the nation's expanding waistline. Excessive weight forces food against the muscle controlling backup. Meanwhile, consumption of fast food plays havoc on the body. You can eat whatever you want occasionally. But a continual diet of the following foods and drinks have been shown to contribute to GERD:

- fatty and fried foods
- citrus fruits and juices
- chocolate
- caffeinated drinks and foods
- excessive alcohol
- garlic and onions
- spicy foods
- tomatoes and tomato-based foods, such as pizza, red spaghetti sauce, and chili
- peppermint and mint flavorings

Baby Talk and Other Resonance Issues

Ever been accused of talking like a baby? Or sounding like you have a perpetual cold or allergy, when you don't? You may be experiencing a problem of resonance. That is the quality of voice that results from how sounds pass through various chambers and cavities.

Try to think of the normal vocal tract like the capital letter *F*.[1] Any interruption of air flow along the letter, such as by placement of the tongue or protruding teeth or blocked cavity, can contribute to a resonance problem. With baby talk, the tongue rises high in the front of the mouth. But what speech therapists call cul de sac resonance results from carrying the tongue high toward the back of the pharynx. This type of sound often comes from deaf speakers. With a nasal sound, the nasal and oral cavities are open. Vowels especially sound like they are coming through the nose. When blockage closes off the two cavities, this produces nasal consonants *m*, *n*, and *j* that sound like you have a stuffed nose.

Most resonance problems stem from too much or too little airflow and sound transmission through the nose. This could be a structural problem, like a cleft palate or abnormal growth. Or resonance differences may result from certain conditions or developmental disorders, such as cerebral palsy. With these conditions,

Ten Ways to Reduce GERD:
Be Your Own Best Advocate

Since most causes of GERD are self-inflicted, there are several things you can do to reduce and prevent symptoms of GERD—and the resulting damage to your voice:

1. Keep a log of what you eat and how your body reacts. Not all foods on the previous list may cause a reaction. But some probably do. By keeping a log or food diary, you can figure out which foods cause the problem. The doctor will be grateful for specific foods and timing that contribute to your condition.

2. Change your diet. Omit trigger foods you discover present a problem.

3. Eat smaller portions. Smaller meals result in less pressure on the esophageal muscle.

4. Limit eating spicy foods.

5. Avoid alcohol and carbonated beverages, both contributors to increased acid.

6. Lose weight if too much is an issue. Check weight charts for guidelines. If excess weight proves a problem, find a weight-loss program that fits your lifestyle choices. And remember to begin or increase exercise to help those good food choices along.

7. Wear loose-fitting clothes. Tight waistbands that squeeze the stomach force food upward. No fun.

8. Stop smoking. Smoking is another major cause of stomach acids acting up.

9. Hold off bedtime for at least two hours after eating to allow digestion to take place.

10. Elevate the head when sleeping. Gravity helps keep the pressure—and digested food—down.

blockage can be effectively reduced or eliminated through surgery or other medical treatments.

In some cases, actors find a nasal voice quality a benefit and choose to continue talking a certain way. Famous actor James Stewart, seen every Christmas in *It's A Wonderful Life*, was able to demonstrate normal resonance, if necessary. But he became known for his nasal drawl. Obviously he saw no need to change his signature voice with so much success. But if he chose to alter how he talked, voice therapy would have led to a reduction of nasal resonance.

Therapy for someone with Stewart's voice quality would emphasize ear training. Then the client could hear normal resonance and correct production of sounds. To monitor success, the therapist might offer audio and video recording devices to play back practice sessions. Such therapy will not necessarily be easy. But with intense practice, improvement will occur.

Noncancerous Vocal Cord Lumps and Bumps

Vocal cord lesions usually develop after trauma to the vocal cords or repeated injury, such as with singers on tour. Pop singers Adele, Keith Urban, and John Mayer have all had painless throat growths that interfered with their singing schedules. Throat lesions can appear in one of three forms, either as polyps, nodules, or cysts. All three cause voice problems, especially for people who rely on their voice for a living. In 2011 Adele wrote on her blog, "My voice yet again went. . . . It just switched off."[2]

Polyps often grow on one side of a vocal fold. They are made up of an outer membrane that encloses a hard mass of tissue. Polyps can appear in different shapes and sizes. The variations influence the type of voice difficulty someone experiences.

Cysts are softer tissue masses also encased in a membrane. They can burrow deeper into the vocal cord or sit near the surface of the fold. Nodules, also called "calluses of the vocal fold,"[3] can arise on either or both sides of vocal cords. They appear wherever there is wearing, much like when new shoes cause a callus on the foot from rubbing when walking. Nodules are hard growths that can lower pitch by preventing vocal folds from normal action. With any lesion, the first line of defense is voice rest, possibly combined with voice therapy. If these cannot alleviate the problem, a doctor may recommend surgery to remove the lesion.

Other Physical Causes

Several conditions can contribute to voice disorders. Vocal folds can freeze and refuse to open and close properly after head, neck, or chest injury, certain

Clues of Vocal Cord Lesions

Lesions on vocal cords can cause a host of problems. Voice differences that may indicate a vocal cord lesion include

- unexpected voice changes,
- low, gravelly voice,
- tired voice,
- low pitch,
- delayed speaking,
- voice cracking,
- breathy voice,
- inability to sing in a high, soft voice,
- unusual effort to speak or sing,
- frequent throat clearing, and
- increased force required to speak.[h]

cancers, thyroid gland problems, or conditions that effect the nervous system. Most diseases of the nervous system that alter the voice occur later in life. But they may appear earlier in a small percentage of young adults. These include stroke (blood clot that interferes with brain function), multiple sclerosis (disease whereby the body attacks its own protective sheath covering nerve fibers and interferes with communication between the brain and rest of the body), or Parkinson's disease (a brain disorder that impairs all organs, including those involved with voice).

The Voice Whisperer

A few people lose their voice altogether, only talking in a whisper. After examination, the doctor may find no physical cause for reduced speaking. Vocal folds work. No bumps or thickening. No underlying illness exists. Then the doctor looks for psychological causes, which may differ with each whisperer.

Well-Known Singer Ends Tour

In 2012, popular songster John Mayer ended his singing tour. His voice sounded scratchy. He felt discomfort and acid reflux. After visiting the doctor, Mayer learned a growth reappeared on the back of his vocal cords, causing his problems. To repair his vocal cords, Mayer underwent a series of throat surgeries. Months of vocal rest, when he wasn't allowed to speak at all, followed each surgery.

"I was forced to type on my iPad to communicate anything," Mayer told an Entertainment TV reporter.[i] Luckily for Mayer's fans, he returned to the touring circuit the next year. This time he was probably a singer more aware of the limits of his voice.

Vocal Fry Trend Spells Disaster

Ever notice how a few reality folks, singers, and actors talk with a low, gravelly voice? Brittany Spears belts out "Oh baby baby" complete with raspy creaks. Same with Kesha. Spears might be projecting this quieter tone to help make her return to higher-range notes easier. Or each singer thinks this way of singing compliments her overheated image. Then there's the Kardashian way of speaking, similarly dropping the voice at the end of sentences.

Reporters noticed that the trend, called vocal fry in professional circles, is catching on with young women everywhere. A 2013 Long Island University study of college women found that two-thirds sounded like they were "running out of oxygen."[j] Another study from the University of Iowa revealed that fluttery, low-pitched voices appeared in an average of 12.5 percent of words uttered by U.S. females, compared with 6.9 percent of Japanese females and 5.6 percent of U.S. males.[k] The way of speaking comes from reduced air flow and prolonged vowel sounds that result from the glottis, or space between the vocal cords, closing. Speech pathologists say this form of vocal abuse may border on a disorder. This is a trend worth passing up.

In some cases, a lost voice simply persists beyond an illness, like a bad habit. In others, a traumatic event, such as a car accident or death, might cause loss of voice. As time passes, the memory and stress of the event lingers long after the trauma occurred. The need to hold onto the whisper or cough or other voice disorder overrides any therapy.

Some people are able to talk normally at certain times, yet produce only strangled sounds at others. When this happens, doctors usually refer the whisperer to a psychologist or psychiatrist. Psychologists look for patterns in when and how someone produces sounds. And doctors work to bring the voice back through gradual behavior therapy to reduce the stress surrounding certain situations.

Taking Care of Your Voice

The voice is a powerful communication tool. You need to treat it kindly to make sure it stays in good working order. Here is what the American Association of Otolaryngologists recommends to prevent voice problems mentioned in this chapter:

- Drink six to eight 8-ounce glasses of water a day. Moisture allows normal secretions to lubricate our vocal cords. If water isn't around, be sure to drink noncaffeinated, nonalcoholic beverages throughout the day.
- Keep screaming or yelling to a minimum. Screaming strains the vocal cord lining.
- Exercise the voice before heavy use, just like you would stretch before heavy exercise or a game. Some exercises include sliding from low to high notes in different vowel sounds, trilling the tongue and lips, or making sounds like a motor boat.
- Never smoke or stop smoking. Smoking inflames vocal cords and can lead to cancer in the larynx, polyps, and a raspy dry voice.
- Practice good breathing techniques. Everyone underestimates how important breathing can be for the entire body. For voice, a good breath fills the lungs before speaking and keeps the flow and strength going.
- Request a microphone before speaking, especially before a large audience or in a large space. A microphone lessens voice strain.
- Be aware of your voice. Stay alert to sudden voice changes. These warn you about a problem that requires modification. Rest the voice. If that doesn't work, and your voice continues to sound different, contact a professional.

Resources

Organizations/Websites

About.com
www.about.com
International physician-written network dedicated to offering targeted medical information to the public, in this case teens. Check out "Teen GERD: What You Need to Know about GERD in Teens," About.com: Heartburn/GERD, heartburn.about.com/od/infantschildrenandreflux/a/teengerdguide.htm

American Academy of Otolaryngology
1650 Diagonal Rd.
Alexandria, VA 22314-2857
1-703-836-4444
www.entnet.org
World's largest organization for specialists who treat ears, nose, throat, head, and neck. The site provides referral and health information for diseases and disorders affecting speech communication.

GI Kids
North American Society for Pediatric Gastroenterology, Hepatology and Nutrition
www.gikids.org/content/27/en/Teen-GERD
Website from an organization of 1,400 pediatric gastroenterologists that offers teens information about how to better understand and improve digestive health, including explaining medical terms and suggestions about how to control GERD.

Health on the Net Foundation
www.healthonnet.org
Site that connects users to specific health information for patients, professionals, and the general public with a separate heading for teens.

Kids Health Info: Voice Disorders
The Royal Children's Hospital
50 Flemington Road Parkville
Victoria 3052 Australia
613-9345-5522
www.rch.org.au/kidsinfo/factsheets.cfm?doc_id=11677
Understandable fact sheets that cover various health issues, including speech and language disorders such as voice disorders.

LiveStrong.com
LiveStrong is a general health and fitness website with a variety of articles. This one is specific to kids and GERD. Check out Julie Boehike, "Heartburn in Children and Pre-teens," LiveStrong.com, August 15, 2011, www.livestrong.com/article/515367-heartburn-in-children-and-pre-teens (accessed July 5, 2013).

Book: Nonfiction

Archuleta, David. *Cords of Strength: A Memoir of Soul, Song, and the Power of Perseverance*. New York: Penguin, 2010. A singer's journey with song and dealing with vocal issues.

WHEN THE BRAIN HEARS AND PROCESSES INFORMATION DIFFERENTLY: LANGUAGE DISORDERS

Famous neurologist and author Oliver Sacks wrote in *The Man Who Mistook His Wife for a Hat*[1] about patients he observed listening to a speech by President Ronald Reagan. As Sacks watched his clients, he noticed something interesting. Several people thought the president's speech was hysterically funny and sat laughing. Others listened stone-faced or looked puzzled. Both groups could hear fine. Yet, they seemed to be listening to different speeches.

Sacks investigated and found that the laughers were patients who had *aphasia*. The condition rendered them unable to understand or express the spoken word. For this group words meant little, so Reagan's words lacked meaning for them. Instead, they focused on the president's body language and tone of voice. These unspoken expressions that go with saying words cannot be faked as easily as quoting words from a speech. The sensitive aphasia group detected a false tone, gesture, and rhythm in the speech that they found comical.

Those who sat without expression or looked puzzled, however, understood the words. But they could not pick up other clues that are part of communication, such as gestures or tone. These people lacked the ability to identify speech that sounded excited, angry, happy, or sad. The patients had what therapists call agnosia. People with agnosia, though they cannot interpret voice quality, can understand grammar involved in presenting a clear and organized speech.

As one patient noted, "Proper words in proper places." This patient said of the speech: "He is not cogent. He does not speak good prose. His word-use is improper. Either he is brain-damaged, or he has something to conceal."[2]

Sure enough, five years after leaving the presidency, Reagan announced that he had Alzheimer's disease, a progressive condition that involves loss of all functions, including the ability to remember, think clearly, and speak. Each group picked up on something unusual in Reagan's presentation. Each displayed one of several language disorders themselves.

What Is a Language Disorder?

For some, a language disorder may appear as a problem with understanding what others say. For others, there may or may not be the same understanding problems, but they may also have difficulty using spoken, written, or symbolic language. Anyone with a language disorder can produce sounds. And their speech is usually understandable. They just lack the ability to make sense of the sounds—either when they are incoming or being produced—and organize their thoughts. Being able to assess language plays a big role in reading and writing.

Language skills are necessary to express needs, ideas, or information. Impaired language indicates challenges with word meaning or how the words sound, such as with fluency or articulation disorders. But those with language disorders do not include young children who merely progress at a slower rate. These children are diagnosed as having delayed language and usually catch up at a later age with children whose language progresses at a regular rate.

Find Something That Allows You to Shine

Making friends can be a challenge for teens with a language disability. People they encounter may shy away from individuals who can't say what they mean or understand what they say. Without the ability to produce or understand regular communication and the body language that goes along with speaking, life can be isolating. That's why parents and therapists encourage teens who have learning challenges to join activities that allow their skills to shine. At the same time, sports, arts, music, or whatever is enjoyable, allows participation in something that doesn't rely on language communication.

A true language disorder shows up as abnormal language development. Adolescents with a language disorder cannot use words in their proper context. The teens may display a defect with expressive language, the ability to express needs. Or problems may result from difficulty with receptive language, impairment in making sense of what others say.

According to the National Dissemination Center for Children with Disabilities, signs of language disorders include the following:

- "improper use of words and their meanings
- inability to express ideas
- inappropriate grammar patterns
- reduced vocabulary
- inability to follow directions"[3]

Problems with language that appear early in life and continue lead to impaired skills with learning in general. The effects go beyond basic written and spoken communication. Many classes, such as history, math, and science, are based on understanding words, concepts, and symbols. If not corrected with speech therapy, language disorders negatively effect later learning, reading, and school achievement in general. Even behavior and social interactions suffer when language cannot be expressed. A language disorder does not mean teens are dumb or cannot learn. It's just that they need to find different ways to understand incoming information and let others know what they grasp.

How Common Are Language Disorders?

Some form of language impairment affects between 6 and 8 million individuals in the United States. This is the largest percentage of communication disorders in the country. A major reason for so many troubles with language comes from the fact that these sorts of challenges can be acquired at any age. And difficulties at different ages develop from many varied causes.

Young children may fail to use language normally from birth. As they mature, they may not acquire or develop language skills that match their age. While many fail to catch up, many more eventually overcome language impairment, usually through therapy. Even children with hearing loss learn to adapt their communication strategies over time.

Adults acquire language disorders from several causes. They may never develop normal language due to mental retardation, autism, or other disorders of brain development. Head injury, stroke, or tumors of the brain can all cause a language disorder at any age that is secondary to the original diagnosis. These

Katy's Story: In Her Own Words

I'm sixteen and a junior in high school. I've had speech therapy growing up because I had difficulty learning and comprehending things. I don't learn fast. I needed repetition a lot of times. On top of that I had a hard time putting words into sentences and comprehending questions.

I didn't realize I had a language problem, but I knew I couldn't read at a young age. A teacher pulled me out of class, but I didn't realize why. The teacher would ask me questions and go over things. We'd play card games with her having cards and asking me to say what was on the cards. Then she'd ask me to make a sentence with each word. These types of activities definitely helped through the years.

I never got bullied, but I never felt as smart as other kids. I was shy because I couldn't read at a young age. I never participated in class. I went along with lessons but never asked questions or told the teacher I didn't understand what was going on. I zoned out a little.

That changed in seventh grade because I had teacher who would read me things and wanted me to summarize what I heard. She asked me questions about what was going on. This special education teacher helped me with memorizing. Something kicked in, and I started to understand.

My original attitude towards speech therapy was I didn't like going because I thought, "What am I doing here: I know these things?" Getting older I know why I'm doing this. I had a disability of not knowing how to read. I do know how to read today: it's improved a lot over before. The therapy has helped a lot.

Now I tell teachers when I need extra help because I don't understand. Sometimes, I get help from special teachers assigned to my class. I also go to a special resource class that's like a study hall. An adult there helps me review my English and history and other work. The support helps me organize. My goals are to improve my reading and comprehension skills, graduate from high school, and go to college, even though entrance exams will be hard. I want to be a journalist.

I think it's okay to admit that you struggle as you learn. It's okay to comprehend things slower than others do, and it's alright to be a visual learner. High school has changed me a lot. I've learned things and matured.[a]

may or may not respond to therapy, or therapy may not be recommended or available.

As with other communication disorders, most studies find more boys than girls with language difficulties. Although estimates vary, ratios can reach two males for every female with a language disorder. Several reasons account for the frequency of language problems with either gender. Some research points to family history. Studies confirm that having an immediate family member with a language or learning challenge increases chances offspring will develop some form of the problem. Research also suggests that having parents with limited education contributes to children developing language difficulties. On the positive side, other studies suggest that breast feeding offsets a lack of parent education and gives a boost to those with language impairment.[4] The jury is still out on specific causes—and prevention—of language disorders.

Researchers do know that damage to different parts of the brain accounts for the type of language disorder someone has. Damage can happen in the part of the brain that produces language or understands language. Or it arises as a result of hearing loss or nerve disorders that interrupt how information is received and produced.

Hearing Loss

So much of how teens learn and express themselves depends upon hearing. Yet, researchers worry that teen hearing loss is close to epidemic proportions. That's bad for communication skills. A 2010 study found that teen hearing loss jumped 31 percent between 1988 and 2006. A whopping one in five U.S. teens between twelve and nineteen years old suffered some hearing loss in 2006. That amounts to about 6.5 million teens, and the numbers keep rising.[5] Ear buds, loud music, even larger and louder concert and sport venues all play a role in the increase of hearing reduction.

Loss or reduction of hearing greatly affects the way teens experience and produce language. As with other communication problems, the earlier and more severe the hearing loss, the more normal development is interrupted. Even mild hearing loss can interfere with language development and success in school, social situations, and jobs. Those affected miss sounds and words. They hear distorted language. They respond to wrong messages. Others may find teens with reduced hearing slow, inattentive, or snobby for not participating in class or social activities. All these communication errors can result from hearing loss. Little do onlookers know that teens with hearing loss are merely trying to mask the fact that they hear less than regular hearing people do.

> ## Teens, Weight, and Hearing Loss
>
> As if there isn't enough bad news about being overweight, a new study of 1,488 boys and girls ages twelve to nineteen found an association between obesity and hearing loss. Teens at or above the 95th percentile on the body mass scale, which measures obesity in humans, are more likely to have poorer hearing over all frequencies. The study revealed almost double the threat of low-frequency loss in at least one ear.
>
> Investigators found no exact cause for the connection. But they suggested that the same inflammation from extra poundage that results in heart and circulation problems may be a factor in damaging hearing apparatus. Just one more reason to keep weight in check.[b]

Hearing loss affects all aspects of daily life. Written English depends upon the spoken word to connect what is spoken with what goes on paper—or computer. Hearing language influences how teens read and comprehend all higher level subjects—from history and science to understanding code systems involved in learning math. Most math and science problems are presented through verbal communication. If hearing is lost or reduced, comprehension, understanding, and problem solving goes, too.

Given these challenges, no wonder studies show that deaf teens who are seventeen or eighteen attain the same literacy level as hearing eight- to nine-year-

> ## Reach Out to Teens with Hearing Loss
>
> "Many teens who are deaf or hard of hearing feel isolated from the hearing world and people around them," said Karena Weil, counselor at the Hearing and Speech Center of North California. "They often struggle with identity issues because they are not 'deaf enough' or 'hearing enough' to feel a sense of belonging. Being a teenager is difficult for all of us. But those with a disability that makes them stand out affects them socially. They really struggle and can be prone to depression, anxiety, and low self-esteem. Often youth with hearing loss feel left out of family functions or conversations."[c] Teens who know someone with a hearing loss need to make an effort to include them in conversation and activities.

olds. These lower test results reflect reduced comprehension skills from hearing loss, rather than lower intelligence. People with hearing loss need to work much harder and for a longer time to reach the same learning goals as other students to get by in school. But complications from hearing loss do not reflect a person's intellectual and career potential.

How We Hear

Hearing disorders arise from two main sources: failure of the hearing system or a breakdown of the nervous system that governs hearing. Many elements contribute to how teens receive, perceive, and understand incoming sounds. The system begins with airwaves from sounds outside the body entering the outer ear. Sound waves travel through delicate middle and inner ear structures on the way to the brain. Inside the brain, these sounds are translated and given meaning, so teens can respond.

Protect Your Hearing

Rock concerts, sporting events, airplanes, loud music—all these and other loud sound producers can affect hearing. So can loud toys, instruments, horns and sirens, and lawn mowers. Any sounds that reach seventy-five decibels or above can harm your hearing, and they seem to be everywhere.

To prevent hearing loss,

- invest in specially designed earmuffs that reduce most sounds to an acceptable level. The National Institute for Occupational Safety and Health estimates that more than fifteen minutes of exposure to 100 decibels or more is unsafe. To get an idea of sound levels, a noisy football stadium can create 100 to 130 decibels. Hearing loss from uncomfortable settings can build over a lifetime without your knowing, so act now.[d]
- buy foam or preformed earplugs that can be found easily in most pharmacies.
- purchase custom-molded plastic or rubber earplugs that are a must for drummers or anyone who attends loud gatherings or mows lawns for extra

cash. Ask for a referral from your ear doctor to find the most reputable specialist.

- avoid loud recreation activities. If you prefer snowmobiling, hunting, or listening to loud music, be sure to wear hearing protectors. Make sure you take breaks from the activity to give your ear mechanisms a rest.
- suggest that your doctor check for ear wax during regular office visits. The shape of some ears encourages more buildup than usual, which requires professional removal. Bad idea to dig deep into the ear yourself. This can cause irreparable damage—and pain.
- use the lowest setting for hair dryers and other appliances that beep or screech—or wear earplugs when using them.
- limit time listening to music through ear buds. Turn volume as low as possible with music, too. Take breaks to give your ears a rest.
- wear earplugs when around noisy machines on the job, including lawn mowers, leaf blowers, and electric drills and saws.

Remember that noise is cumulative and can injure your ears unless they are properly protected.

More specifically, sound waves into the outer ear move through the ear canal toward the *eardrum*, also known as the tympanic membrane. The sensitive eardrum causes a series of bones on the other side to vibrate, resulting in a pattern of sound waves. These tiny bones comprise the *middle ear*. Once incoming waves reach the middle ear, the bones pulsate and enhance the sound waves, which sends them into the fluid-filled inner ear.

Tiny hairs line the inner ear. Fluid in the *inner ear* moves these miniature hairs. Movement translates the sound waves into nerve impulses that travel inside the brain. Any breakdown in this process can create a hearing loss. An estimated 1.9 percent of school-aged children and teens experience reduced hearing in one or both ears.[6]

Sounds are measured in units called decibels. The higher the number of decibels, the louder the noise. Sounds from the environment usually range between 30 and 80 decibels. For example, busy traffic measures about 80 decibels, and regular conversation clocks in at 60 decibels. But hearing a lawn mower at 90 decibels, rock music at 110 decibels, a jet plane at 120 decibels, or firecrackers at

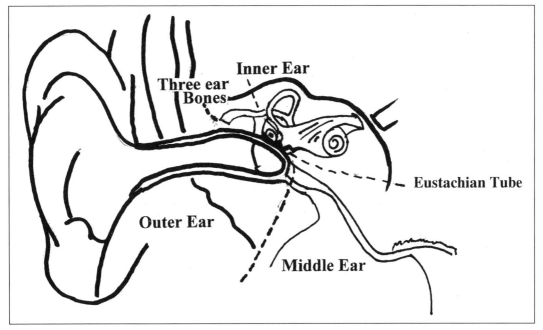

Anatomy of the human ear. *Illustration by Anne Ryan.*

Joys and Dangers of Cell Phones

Sure cell phones are convenient, accessible, and fun to use. But not all is positive in cell phone land. Sometimes, danger comes from good things. Much of the danger with mobile phones lies in driving while talking. Research from University of Utah psychologists found that drivers who talk on any device—handheld or hands free—are equally impaired while driving. In fact, they can be as dangerous as legally drunk drivers. Distractions include manipulating a handheld phone while steering, shifting gears, and using turn signals. They also involve the conversation itself, which distracts from focusing on the road. Specific study results found talking drivers hit the brakes 9 percent slower, exhibited 24 percent more variation in distance between cars as attention changed between driving and talking, were 19 percent slower to resume speed after braking, and were more likely to rear-end the car in front of them. An earlier study discovered that teens and young adults who drive while talking on cell phones had the same slow reaction time as senior drivers.[e]

140 decibels can harm your hearing. The longer your exposure above 85 decibels lasts, the greater your chance of severe hearing loss.[7]

Conductive Hearing Loss

The most common *conductive hearing losses* come from colds, allergies, or infection. These can cause fluid to build up in the middle ear. With nowhere to go, the fluid blocks airwaves from normal passing into the inner ear, therefore limiting or totally blocking hearing. Sometimes, mild infections cause buildup that cannot be identified as a problem. Or teens refuse to admit that allergies are affecting their hearing. Only when distorted sounds or repeated requests from others to talk louder become a disturbing pattern, do hearing-impaired teens investigate further.

In young children, chronic ear infections can contribute to slower language development. With school-age children and adults, infections can interrupt all sorts of learning and social activities. Communication sounds distorted. Words that are heard don't make sense. Therefore, finding a medical remedy early is important.

Most infections can be treated with medicine. In cases of continual ear infections, some doctors recommend surgery to place tubes in the eardrum to keep pathways clear. The surgery may require anesthetic to either freeze the area or induce sleep, but the procedure is usually pain free afterward. Tubes pop out any time from a few months to years later. In the meantime, tubes allow ears—and hearing—to heal from constant infection.

Sometimes, conductive hearing losses develop due to malformed parts of the outer or middle ears. One example is otosclerosis, which does not appear until the teen years. With otosclerosis, a growth develops surrounding bones of the middle ear. This inhibits their vibrating, thus interrupting their ability to receive and move sound waves. Usually, this form of conductive impairment can be treated successfully by surgery.

Nerve or Sensory Hearing Loss

Hearing loss due to loss of nerve sensations often produces greater and more permanent communication problems than conductive losses. Nerve loss can appear at any age. Babies can be born with nerve hearing loss if the mother contracted an infection, such as measles or mumps, or the baby experienced a lack of oxygen during delivery. Heredity plays a role, if parents have a history of hearing loss.

When hearing ever suddenly disappears, run to the doctor. Sudden hearing loss can happen at any time. Those affected may wake up with severely reduced or no hearing. Or they notice quickly diminishing hearing within minutes or over one or two hours. The abrupt loss can occur in one or both ears, although sudden loss rarely happens in both ears. Severe loss often comes with a whooshing sound, like rushing water or annoying ringing in the ear. Without warning, teens can lose their ability to receive incoming messages, which interferes with communicating. They may feel off balance or dizzy.

This type of loss results from damage to the auditory nerve. Doctors call this *sudden sensorineural hearing loss*, or nerve deafness in lay terms. In 1 to 3 percent of cases, a brain tumor is involved. But tumors on the auditory nerve that controls

Guns and Hearing Loss

Let others debate the pros and cons about who should use guns and when and where. Many Americans find this is an emotional issue. What isn't emotional but fact is firearms produce loud noise. And that noise causes hearing problems, if the shooters refuse to protect their ears.

The American Speech-Language-Hearing Association claims that noise louder than 140 decibels can damage hearing, often forever. Now consider that different firearms reach sound bursts of between 145 and 175 decibels. If shooters are enclosed in a place with solid walls or add devices to modify their weapon, sound levels can climb considerably higher.

Hearing loss that is mild affects high frequencies. This type of loss causes trouble hearing high-pitched sounds, such as the letters *s*, *v*, or *th*. Someone with an undetected loss may accuse others of mumbling or hear ringing in the ears. The ear closest to the gun will experience greater loss. But hearing loss can worsen over time, sometimes to the point of deafness.

If you must shoot firearms, the best thing to do is protect your ears with thick muffs, earplugs, or both. Hunters who worry about hearing approaching game should invest in special hearing devices that soften sounds but still allow them to hear. Reducing hearing when hunting is a small price to pay when life-long total hearing is at stake.

hearing are rare. Doctors have offered several theories about what else destroys nerve cells that affect hearing. These theories look into severe infections, head trauma, stroke, and some antibiotics. But none are the final word.

When hearing suddenly disappears, seek medical assistance immediately. The reason is this form of sensory hearing loss can be repaired. On occasion hearing returns on its own. But loss can become permanent if not dealt with within twenty-four to forty-eight hours.

The doctor will either recommend that you see an otolaryngologist or prescribe medication without referral. Taking appropriate medication within one to two days usually restores hearing. Without immediate medication, hearing may never return, as the nerve cannot be repaired once it dies.

Improving Language with Impaired Hearing

When hearing loss is great, many families opt for separate education for the deaf, the most extreme situation. These individuals may rely on sign language, a universal way of communicating through a system of hand signals. Within an environment where everyone communicates in sign language, someone with hearing loss can participate fully. But sign language can be socially limiting. Someone who speaks this way can only communicate with others who know sign language.

In the hearing community, however, social isolation from peers and family can be a huge problem with hearing loss. The opportunity to communicate, socialize, and learn becomes limited. As a result, many teens with hearing loss who remain in the hearing community feel depressed about being different. Hearing loss contributes to low self-esteem, which further limits the desire to interact.

New electronic devices have been a boon for people with hearing problems. In past years, teens might have been embarrassed to be seen in public with headphones and gadgets coming out of their ears. In this era of technology advances,

Celebrate Better Hearing and Speech Month

The American Speech-Language-Hearing Association (ASHA) believes communication is so important that it created Better Hearing and Speech Month. Each May since 1927, ASHA publicizes its national campaign to raise awareness of communication disorders. Part of the program emphasizes the importance of prevention and treatment of hearing loss. To learn more about Better Hearing and Speech Month and how you can promote it in your school and community, check out www.asha.org/bhsm.

it's trendy. Eyeglass hearing aids, behind the ear hearing aids, inside the ear hearing aids. Those teens with hearing challenges now fit into the crowd. What are the differences between hearing aids and other enhanced listening or music devices?

Many devices that augment hearing and communication are becoming more readily available. Teletypewriters (TTYs) and telephone instruments specifically

Tips for Boosting Language with Hearing Loss

- Tell others which ear hears better than the other, if loss is in one ear. Friends and family are kind about speaking on the hearing side, if they know.
- Try to stay clear of noisy environments, if you use a hearing aid. Many aids magnify all sounds, which makes focusing on conversation difficult.
- Explain to others they don't need to shout because you have hearing loss.
- Text or use computers to convey messages, when appropriate.
- Adjust to a hearing aid by going to an audiologist trained in fitting and troubleshooting proper positioning, control adjustments, and caring for the device.
- Choose less crowded times to eat out.
- Request a table against a wall or in a booth and away from the kitchen or staging area where dishes clatter in a restaurant.
- Use visual cues when speaking with someone else. Think about facial expression, body language, and context to make sense of what is being said.
- Face the person you are speaking with to help you focus on what that person is saying, even if you do not read lips. Good eye contact is important with any conversation, whether or not hearing loss is involved.
- Install visual cues, such as a blinking light, to alert you when the phone or doorbell is ringing. Put the cell phone on vibrate.
- Learn how to ask for assistance. Ask people to rephrase, if you cannot understand what they say. Most folks are accommodating, if they know someone doesn't understand.

for the deaf (TTDs) give teens with severe hearing loss the ability to communicate language over long distances. Computers take this ability to a whole different level. They equalize the communication experience and take hearing and speaking out of the interaction completely.

Other options for severe hearing loss involve hearing aids and surgery for cochlear implants. While hearing aids amplify sounds, a cochlear implant converts sound waves to electrical pulses. These pulses stimulate the nerve to heighten perceptions. Cochlear implants do not restore hearing: they merely enhance the ability to sense sounds. The idea is this ability allows someone with severe hearing loss to better participate in the hearing world. Different groups pose pros and cons about the benefits and drawbacks of this route to enhanced language skills.

Learning Disabilities

The more likely language disorder that you will encounter—either for yourself or someone you know—is a *learning disability*. The term *learning disabilities* actually covers several disorders of brain structure that influence learning. Language is a major component of learning disabilities, although other areas of learning can be affected. The disorder results from a difference in how a person's brain is wired. Someone with a learning disability may have trouble in language areas of reading, writing, spelling, reasoning, and organizing information. They have different learning styles that need to be understood before learning can take place. Some teens learn better by listening, while others understand through visual cues. But they are just as smart—or smarter—than peers.

Learning disabilities encompass one of the most common childhood disorders. By school age, teachers find that almost 7 percent of students have a learning disability that would benefit from special learning techniques.[8]

Learning disabilities and differences in the brain are present at birth. Usually they arise as a result of heredity, running in families. Studies indicate that between 20 and 40 percent of learning disabilities are inherited from another family member.[9] The disability can be specific to language or related to learning in general. Unlike some speech and language disorders, learning disabilities are lifelong. But with therapy, support services, and accommodations, teens with learning disabilities can do anything.

The term *learning disability* does not include individuals with particular emotional disturbances, limited intellect, or impaired senses, which is an important distinction. People with learning disabilities are not dumb or automatic trouble. That said, teens who have learning disabilities may experience more challenges with learning than average students. These may contribute to seeming bored, acting out, or feeling badly about themselves at times, particularly in school.

Twelve Well-Known People with Learning Disabilities

Learning disabilities can be challenging, but they do not have to be a handicap. You know more people than you think who have not only conquered living with a learning disability but thrived.[f]

Avi, author of more than seventy books for children and young adults, who failed every class in high school before his parents enrolled him in a private school where he learned to read and write

Cher, singer/entertainer who couldn't remember numbers or balance a checkbook

Tom Cruise, actor who still learns his lines by listening to tapes because he has dyslexia

Walt Disney, cartoonist, movie producer, and creator of the Disney entertainment empire who was thought a slow learner as a child

Thomas Edison, inventor of the light bulb and phonograph whose family thought him dumb and troublesome

Albert Einstein, physicist who didn't talk until age four or read until age nine and who failed college entrance exams, yet his mind conquered scientific worlds unheard of earlier

Richard Engle, NBC foreign correspondent whose learning disabilities give him extra energy to tour the globe to search for a good story

Jay Leno, comedian and talk show host who frequently mentions how he mixes up words because he has dyslexia

Patricia Palocco, children's book author and illustrator who told her story about struggling to learn to read in her book *Thank You Mr. Falkner.*

George Patton, World War II general who couldn't read until he was twelve years old and passed through school by memorizing rather than reading

Nelson Rockefeller, former vice president and wealthy businessman who was thought dull until age nine because he didn't know the alphabet

Stan Wattles, Indy race car driver who found racing around a track doesn't require reading

Stuart's Story: In His Own Words

Dyslexia for me, it's about reading, penmanship, and the ability to write at all. My brain has no way to put down what I'm trying to say. Even something as ordinary as filling out a check can be awful. I'd fill out numbers and my name before I went anywhere. On some days, I couldn't write my signature. It's a coordination of brain, mind, and eye. Now I use credit cards.

When I was little, I'd feel frustrated and confused. I had scrambled visual signals. In school, I needed to use visual signals that wouldn't come. So I flunked a grade. I went through school feeling tremendous shame, embarrassment, and self-consciousness because I couldn't read. I became antisocial. I wouldn't let anyone come to my house. I walked hunched over because I believed I deserved to be punished. My mother said one day she saw me leaning against the wall at school and not playing with anyone at recess. She cried all the way home.

A psychologist sent me to military school, where I learned to be tough. After that, going to high school was easy. I was able to meet new friends, who didn't know about my not being able to read. I was free from the stigma.

I can see a general outline or pattern of things but not the things themselves. I adapted to reading by memorizing the lengths and shapes of words. I used visual cues the way a Chinese person might learn a pictograph. I never became a good student in high school, but I bloomed. By then, I had memorized tens of thousands of words by their shape and other cues.

I was good at conceptualizing. I could pick up on mannerisms before words. When I'm reading someone's comment on Facebook, I have to read four or five times to make sense of it. Maybe I need the body language, which you don't get with written words. Straight words don't help me interpret my environment. But my handwriting is good on the computer.

I found out I had dyslexia in college. I was asked to read a paragraph, and I couldn't. I also have problems of turning thoughts into words. People on the Internet say my writing sounds awkward. It's coordinating the speech with my fingers that doesn't work, although I'm a thoughtful thinker. And interestingly, I can paint and sculpt, probably because the materials dictate what comes out. But I'm glad to have a name to what I have, so I don't feel so much of an outcast.[9]

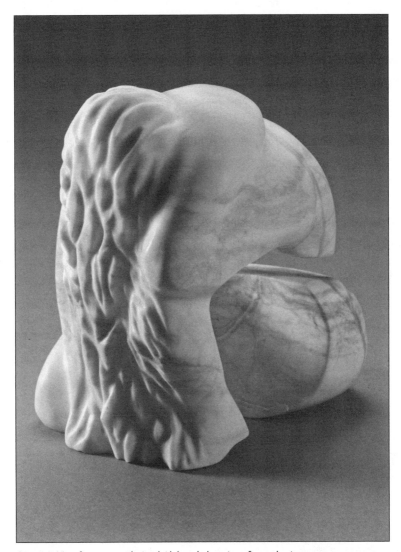

Stuart Kaufman sculpted this alabaster female to convey a message of sadness that goes unseen behind a mask of hair. *Courtesy of artist Stuart Kaufman.*

Dyslexia

According to the American Speech-Hearing-Language Association, another name for language-based learning disability is *dyslexia*. Dyslexia is actually a cluster of symptoms that involve difficulties with language. The disorder shows up when any reading, spelling, and writing skills fall below the same age level as with peers.[10] Other aspects of learning may be normal or superior. But anything involving language proves particularly problematic. Recognizing words, sounding out letters and symbols, reading aloud, spelling, writing essays, following grammar rules, sometimes just trying to talk—all these can be challenging, depending upon how mild or severe the dyslexia. About 80 percent of students with a learning disability have problems with reading, many that are lifelong.

Some teens with dyslexia may mix up words when talking, such as saying "tomorrow" when meaning "yesterday." Others may forget or mix up letters when writing, such as printing "d" for "b" as in "deb" for "bed." Or they may confuse word order, for example, "Let's outside go." Or confuse left and right. Reversals, substitutions, and omissions and additions of words and letters are common with dyslexia. Trouble summarizing, grasping abstract concepts, focusing on details too much or too little, or completing open-ended questions on tests are all indications that a learning disability may be present.

School can be a nightmare when dyslexia is involved. Remembering and managing symbols extends to trouble with math. Homework instructions are unreadable, let alone understandable. Schedules, due dates, and managing time can be overwhelming when someone cannot understand what needs to be accomplished.

Improving Communication with Dyslexia

Because teens with dyslexia have trouble expressing themselves, they may have trouble beyond the classroom. Work, dating, and relating at home can all be minefields. But there are things that can be done to make life easier.[h]

- Get a diagnosis early. Make sure other overlapping problems, such as attention deficit disorder (ADD) or attention-deficit/hyperactivity disorder (ADHD), aren't interfering with treatment plans.
- Find a good speech and language therapist who understands dyslexia.
- Build on strengths for confidence and an eye toward a possible career.
- Remediate weaknesses, which involves a ton of persistence.
- Practice reading strategies, both oral and silent reading. Memorize sight words. Learn sounds for letters and letter-sound groups. Develop comprehension strategies that fit your form of dyslexia. Look for clues in pictures or other visuals that can help reveal meaningful content. And practice, practice, practice.

- Ask for help when you cannot understand something or need special accommodations at school. Request extra time to complete tests or projects, if slow reading is a problem. Ask for someone to read instructions to you. Request a waiver from foreign language, if language processing presents difficulties. Asking is *not* a weakness: it is a way to improve.
- Record class/work discussions, if listening is a better way to learn. Find books on tape and recorded textbooks. Record reports and essays first, and transcribe them once they have been composed.
- Establish a regular time for homework to avoid procrastination and encourage organization. Work in a set part of the house, and have supplies ready to use. Keep separate supplies and books at home and at school to limit problems that result from forgetting these items.
- Use a laptop computer, if handwriting is illegible. Ask the teacher if you could use a computer to take notes and for homework or to ask questions after school hours. Use PowerPoint to guide oral reports. Download apps and an online dictionary to help with spelling, grammar, and writing. Listen to the playback voice feature, if the computer has one.
- Borrow notes from someone else, even the teacher.
- Watch people for clues about what they are saying, if listening to words is confusing. Hand gestures, loudness, and facial features can all be clues to meaning.
- Check out colleges offering programs that provide remedial work and support. There are no required Individualized Education Programs in college, so students are on their own, unless they can hook into a support system on campus. Libraries and school counselors have college catalogs of institutions that offer learning and studying assistance.
- Join a support group at school, at a community center, or through an organization or speech center that invites teens with similar problems to meetings. Support groups confirm you are not alone in the journey with learning disabilities.
- Never expect changes overnight. Look to conquering symptoms of dyslexia over the long haul.

Seven Things Someone with a Learning Disability or Autism Hates to Hear

Next time you want to say any of these statements to someone, think again and don't. They can be hurtful—and they are not helpful.

1. Try harder.
2. Your future is toast if you can't learn to read and write.
3. This is easy.
4. Get your act together and organize yourself.
5. You're not focusing.
6. Can't you ever finish anything you start?
7. Act your age.

Teens with dyslexia work slower, if at all. They pay attention to details, rather than get the main points. They have trouble summarizing and outlining. Dyslexia may mean working harder and longer, but it doesn't mean teens are not creative, industrious, and able to learn.

Autism

Autism is another disability that may result in serious language challenges. The condition can range from mild to severe, which is what professionals call *autism spectrum disorder*. The most common signs of autism involve language and communication and social skills.

Each marker along the spectrum indicates how someone communicates and interacts with others. Someone with mild autism, also called Asperger's syndrome, may be able to communicate but in an awkward manner. Someone with severe autism may grunt or point or scream instead of speaking.

Communication develops differently for many people with autism. Whereas nondisabled children usually understand more than they express, a child with autism may exhibit reverse skills. Or they may seem to fluctuate in this ability. One day they say more than they understand. On another they may understand yet not respond to regular conversation.

An early sign of autism is the failure to develop usable language. Some parents first notice symptoms at birth, such as trouble suckling or a lack of eye contact.

John's Story Growing Up with Autism: In His Own Words

I remember I went to special schools and had speech therapy. I was frustrated and would bite my hand. At about six-and-a-half, I talked in sentences and could count. I used to throw fits, but I don't remember why. When I misbehaved, I had to go to a corner in my room. I was hyper but outgrew that by sixth grade. I still deal with frustration today. I'm dating a girl, and I yell at her—but not [yell] at work.

My parents had faith in me, and I wanted to prove I could do better. I didn't want to settle for low classes in high school. I think you should give kids motivation and be patient. They will show what they can do. If parents could just spend time, it could work out. I heard from my mother that she spent a lot of time with me.

I used to talk to myself a lot. I had an imaginary family and would go through scenarios. They were wonderful stories where I'd put myself in their shoes or daydream into the future. Guess I was blocking out the world. As years went by, the imaginary family went away. But the stories didn't stop until I was twenty-seven, when I moved into an apartment. I guess these stories were a stress reliever.

Loud sounds bother me. I like music soft. At rock concerts, I used to stick cotton and fingers in my ears and still didn't like it. One thing that fascinated me was ringing ears. When I go to sleep I use classical music to softly drown out the ringing in my ears.

When I was a camp counselor, campers and counselors treated me badly. As a teen I was bothered because I was ignored. I would have loved to not be picked on as much, called names, or ignored. My older brother didn't understand me until years later. He always looked at me as odd.

If I knew someone was starting a new job, I would tell people at the work to say "hi," "welcome," and introduce themselves. I want people to tell me short cuts about how to succeed. When you go for a job interview, ask for an application, be on time, don't wear sunglasses or shorts, comb your hair and look nice, talk in complete sentences, and have good grammar. And that's it.[i]

More commonly, parents worry something is wrong around the time babies usually begin talking. A baby with autism may start babbling and cooing but with a smaller range of sounds than a child without autism. Or they may squeal instead, which can be a trial for family members or others around them. Even when a child begins uttering a few words, these may suddenly stop. Parents and doctors usually take a wait-and-see attitude, at least until the baby reaches about age two or three. The lack of language becomes more obvious, which signals a problem. Then doctors recommend a more in-depth evaluation.

Although autistic behaviors range from mild to severe and can change and improve over time, language difficulties persist into adulthood, even with Asperger's syndrome. Language can be grunts or relatively normal-sounding. Teens with autism who remain nonverbal need to live and work in situations with supervision. With Asperger's, individuals can eventually function independently and speak regularly. Moreover, they may test well in school yet lack common sense and street smarts that understanding and using language requires. But they miss social cues, such as when they are talking too much or too loud or when others stop listening. And they lack other behaviors, for example, eye contact, that go along with participating in a conversation.

Autism Doesn't Stop Dreaming—and Succeeding

In high school, Alexis Wineman realized she was her parents' fourth child, which meant money for college would be tight by the time she graduated. When Alexis's mother suggested entering a beauty pageant to earn money, Ms. Wineman never figured her daughter would find that a good idea. Alexis has autism.

Her condition is so high level, though, that she wasn't diagnosed until she was age eleven. Until then, Alexis just felt different and wanted other kids to stop making fun of her. Now she embraces the diagnosis, just as she embraced the idea of competing.

Alexis sometimes "struggles to communicate" and often takes things too literally.[j] Still, she managed to win the Miss Montana title. That win secured her place in the final 2013 Miss America pageant. At age eighteen, Alexis became the youngest contestant and the only one with autism. The teen, who communicated in concrete terms, had a secret weapon no one anticipated. For the talent portion of the competition, Alexis performed a stand-up comedy routine, one on body image. Although she didn't win the contest, Alexis became a profound voice for the potential of individuals with disabilities.

When speaking, their voices sound flat and without varied pitch or emotion. Words are expressed in a mechanical manner. Conversations focus on concrete, straightforward topics or fixate on one topic that is of special interest. Teachers sometimes first spot higher functioning children with autism who have never been identified by how their communication lacks understanding of abstract concepts. Some believe that Asperger's syndrome is a separate condition from autism, but they are closely linked in their problems with using language.

Currently one out of every eight children show signs of autism. Incidence of autism continues to rise, but researchers are unsure why. Investigations uncovered several causes for the condition and its increase. So far, a mix of genetic and environmental causes seems likely. Twin studies have confirmed several genes that may trigger symptoms. Scans show differences in brains of individuals with and without autism. One theory suggests that genes play a role in how the brain develops and how brain chemicals interact. Other theories look at environmental factors, such as air quality, foods, or immunizations.[11]

So far, nothing has surfaced as the exact cause, and no treatment makes autism disappear. The best treatment is early education that focuses on specific language and social skills that people with autism cannot pick up naturally. Fortunately, learning these skills can be lifelong, showing constant improvement.

Temple Grandin Speaks for Autistics Who Cannot

Listening to Temple Grandin, an animal scientist, give a bookstore presentation in about 1998 proved an interesting experience. Before Grandin spoke, the bookseller cautioned the audience not to clap, as loud sounds upset her. The woman told people to ask questions after raising a hand and in a quiet manner. She said Grandin wouldn't look at us when she signed books. And never, ever try to shake her hand, as touch bothered her, too. As the speech unfolded, Grandin's responses, while informative and intelligent, sounded canned and mechanical. That was because Temple Grandin has autism, something she researches, writes, and speaks about often.

Grandin and the book she was promoting gave insight into why adults with autism act a certain way. She told of her childhood and how she failed to understand and be understood by her classmates. She explained her silent fears of certain overwhelming sounds, touch, and smells, and daydreams that interfered with learning and interacting,

I think in pictures. Words are like a second language to me. I translate both spoken and written words into full-color movies, complete with sounds, which run like a tape in my head. When somebody speaks to me, the words are instantly translated into pictures. Language-based thinkers, those who learn by listening rather than visually, often find this phenomenon difficult to understand. But in my job as an equipment designer for the livestock industry, visual thinking is a tremendous advantage. Visual thinking has enabled me to build entire systems in my imagination.

One of the most profound mysteries of autism has been the remarkable ability of most autistic people to excel at visual spatial skills while performing so poorly at verbal skills. When I was a child and teenager, I thought everybody thought in pictures. I had no idea that my thought processes were different. In fact, I did not realize the full extent of the differences until very recently. At meetings I started asking other people detailed questions about how they accessed information from their memories. From their answers I learned that my visualization skills far exceeded those of most other people.[k]

When asked if she would rather not be autistic, Grandin replied, "I like the way I think. I like logical thinking."[l]

Years later during another interview, Grandin made eye contact. She now talked with animation and body language. The interviewer asked Grandin if characteristics of autism can ever be modified and controlled. She said simply, "I am living proof that they can."[m]

Teens with autism, especially those individuals who are lower functioning, may be unable to comprehend and express themselves to satisfy their needs. They may create their own language, substituting words or letters to say what only they understand. Teens with autism may leave out words or letters when talking. They often cannot control the pitch and loudness of their voice.

Since many people with autism have difficulty processing information through their senses, too little or too much of what they hear, feel, or see can cause them to overreact or underreact. Painful sensations may result in their becoming withdrawn or silent and unresponsive. Or they may throw tantrums or scream to block out disturbing sounds, smells, touch, sights, or movements.

Many teens at the higher functioning range of autism find they cannot understand any language taken out of context. They think in a very concrete, straight-

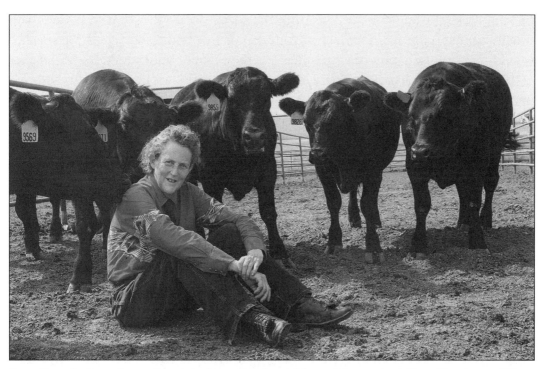

Teen Temple Grandin easily related to animals and found they calmed her. *Courtesy of Temple Grandin.*

forward way. They often cannot grasp two definitions of the same word or how a word or phrase may actually mean something else on a different occasion. As an example, sayings like "hungry as a horse" may prompt someone with autism to turn around looking for the horse. Or "use a little elbow grease" might send them to a mirror to check their elbows.

Autistic language often mimics what others have said in word, pitch, and tone but without understanding of meaning. Some teens with autism repeat commercials or, in the olden days, names and addresses from the telephone book. Or they repeat words, phrases, or sentences, even in settings where they make no sense. A good example is the 1988 movie *Rain Man*. In this movie actor Tom Cruise plays a young man who suddenly discovers he has a brother, Raymond, played by Dustin Hoffman. Hoffman is a high-functioning autistic who repeats names and addresses from the telephone book.

Other people with autism may answer questions by repeating what has been asked but curiously changing pronouns. For example, "Do you want to go with me to a movie?" is asked, but the response may be "Do me want to go to a movie?" Still other teens fixate on one topic, often becoming experts. They engage everyone they meet with the minute details of a legal case or investigation into how light travels through a lamp.

Another hallmark of autistic language is the inability to handle back-and-forth conversations that come so easily to most teens. This develops from difficulty picking up subtle and correct cues from the social world. People who have autism usually cannot judge from someone's tone of voice or body language if the speaker is kidding, serious, happy, or angry. Because they cannot understand the social cues of language, much like someone with agnosia, they do not know how to respond in a manner that fits the discussion. As a result, interactions may seem awkward or filled with uncomfortable pauses. This is when someone with autism chooses to fill the conversation void by repeating a song or commercial.

Children with autism who develop usable language by age five usually have brighter futures. But with autism the sky's the limit, if proper language therapy comes early and often. There is no magic cutoff, as everyone keeps learning, whether in school or not. One student first gained usable language when he was twelve years old and gradually added social communication over the following years.[12] John began talking when he was six years old. With intense therapy and family support, he went on to attain a college degree and live and work independently.

Twelve Ways to Improve Language with Autism

If you know someone with autism,

- constantly talk about what the person with autism is doing, as the activities occur. This communication models language and its organization.
- review what the teen has done and will do. Focusing on real-world discussions keeps the person with autism from veering into talk about fixations.
- encourage participation in new experiences to expand language and vocabulary. Varied activities allow someone with autism to feel more comfortable in different social situations.
- play board games, so the person with autism learns how to take turns and that games and social interactions have rules.

If you have autism,

- read books aloud with someone to hear how sentences are organized.
- read into a tape recorder to hear back how your voice sounds. Practice reading words in higher or lower voices or with different emphasis to sound less robotic. Underline words to help you remember to emphasize them.

- talk in front of a mirror to see how to increase body language that accompanies vocal language.
- connect with others on the computer. These interactions happen without eye contact or the need for body language or voice inflection, making socializing easier. Remember to request adult supervision to make sure you are on safe websites.
- listen to stories to hear how letter sounds turn into words and sentences.
- watch movies to see how actors show different expressions.
- read the same article or book as a friend or family member. Talk about what you read together. What are the highlights of the story? What wasn't understood? Tell them to ask you questions.
- sing to convey information. Singing provides a role model for sound production that can improve articulation as well as socialization.

Resources

Organizations/Websites

Alexander Graham Bell Association for the Deaf and Hard of Hearing
3417 Volta Place, NW
Washington, DC 20007
202-337-5220 (voice); 202-337-5221 (TTY)
nc.agbell.org
Information center about technology, support, and advocacy for families and professionals involved with hearing loss.

American Society for Deaf Children
3820 Hartzdale Drive
Camp Hill, PA 17011
866-895-4206 (voice)
717-334-7922 (voice/TTY)
www.deafchildren.org
A national organization that supports and educates families and professionals who connect with children and teens with hearing loss and deafness.

Autism Society
www.autism-society.org
Oldest national autism resource.

Center for Hearing and Communication
50 Broadway, 6th Floor
New York, NY 10004
917-305-7700 (voice)
917-305-7999 (TTY)
www.chchearing.org
Organization that offers people of all ages who are hard of hearing or deaf diag-
nostic, counseling, rehabilitation, and education programs regardless of how they
communicate.

Dyslexia My Life, Girard Sagmiller
www.dyslexiamylife.org
Website founded by Girard Sagmiller, award-winning advocate, motivational
speaker, and author of *Dyslexia My Life* for individuals with dyslexia and other
learning disabilities.

Hearing Loss Association of America
7910 Woodmont Avenue, Suite 1200
Bethesda, MD 20814
301-657-2248 (voice/TTY)
www.hearingloss.org
A national support and resource network of fourteen state organization and 200 local
chapters that helps people with learning loss and their families live with hearing loss.

International Dyslexia Association
40 York Road, 4th Floor
Baltimore, MD 21204
800-ABCD-123
410-296-0232
www.interdys.org
Organization dedicated to helping individuals with dyslexia and their families
through conferences, newsletters, research, and professional referrals.

Learning Disabilities Association of America
4156 Library Road
Pittsburgh, PA 15234-1349
412-341-1515

www.ldaamerica.org
Largest organization advocating for individuals with learning disabilities with local centers in forty-two states. Each provides services and support, including a journal, to people with learning disabilities of different ages in all aspects of their lives.

National Center for Disease and Disabilities
www.cdc.gov/ncbddd/autism/index.html
National web page about autism spectrum disorder that is prepared by the Center for Disease Control.

National Center for Learning Disabilities
381 Park Avenue South, Suite 1401
New York, NY 10016
888-575-7373
www.ncld.org
Information, resources, and advocacy center for anyone dealing with learning disabilities.

Temple Grandin
www.templegrandin.com
Temple Grandin's website with considerable information about autism and animal behavior. There is also an "Ask Temple!" section for questions, which she will answer.

Books: Nonfiction

Cook O'Toole, Jennifer. *The Asperkids (Secret) Book of Social Rules: The Handbook of Not-So-Obvious Social Guidelines for Tweens and Teens with Asperger Syndrome*. New York: Jessica Kingsley Publishing, 2012.
Montgomery, Sy. *Temple Grandin: How the Girl Who Loved Cows Embraced Autism and Changed the World*. Boston: Houghton Mifflin Books for Children, 2012. Thorough biography for adolescent readers about Temple Grandin growing up with autism.
Mooney, Jonathon, and Cole, David. *Learning Outside the Lines: Two Ivy League Students with Learning Disabilities and ADHD Give You the Tools for Academic Success and Educational Revolution*. New York: Simon & Schuster, 2000.
Schultz, Philip. *My Dyslexia*. New York: W.W. Norton and Company, 2012. Thought-provoking memoir about Schultz's journey through life with dyslexia from his early troubles learning to read to becoming an award-winning poet.

Taylor, John. *Kids with ADD and ADHD*. Minneapolis, MN: Free Spirit Press, 2006. Information and advice for teens with different learning styles that cover everyday topics, such as getting a job, planning for the future, dating, driving, and knowing your rights with education laws and with interpersonal relationships.

Book: Fiction

Betancourt, Jeanne. *My Name Is Brian*. New York: Scholastic, 1995. Story about a sixth grader with dyslexia who covers his embarrassment about his trouble reading and writing by being the class clown.

DVD

Jackson, Mick, dir. *Temple Grandin*. HBO Home Video, 2010. HBO movie about the life and successes of Temple Grandin, who has autism.

Levinson, Barry, dir. *Rain Man*. MGM, 1988. Award-winning movie with Dustin Hoffman as a high-functioning young man with autism who is suddenly taken from the institution where he lived by actor Tom Cruise, who never knew he had a brother before his parents died or what autism was.

CARS, GUNS, SPORTS, AND THE UNEXPECTED: BRAIN INJURY AND COMMUNICATION

....

What do cars, guns, and sports have to do with language? Plenty, at least when brain injuries from any of these things occur. As a teenager you don't expect any harm to come to you—any time, for any reason. In fact, you probably assume you are practically invincible, unless maybe you are the kind of person who is obsessed with news, action films, or video games that thrive on shoot-em-up bad events happening. But terrible things *can* happen, many that are beyond your control.

Traumatic Brain Injury

The American Medical Association refers to traumatic brain injury (TBI) as any physical injury caused by an outside force, such as an automobile accident, or an internal problem, such as a growth.[1] Any part of the body can be hurt by trauma, but head injuries cause the greatest changes to speech, language, thinking, emotion, and overall communication. Resulting damage can be temporary or lasting, even fatal.

A TBI does not come from heredity, birth trauma, or a degenerative disease. But it can result from a blow, jolt, or bump to the head that is strong enough to disrupt normal functioning. Disruptions can be as mild as a headache to a severe enough assault to cause loss of memory or consciousness, as Shannon faced (see Shannon's Story on page 106). Luckily, three out of four brain injuries are mild.

Shannon's Story: In Her Own Words

I left my dorm with new college friends to drive to a party. We passed a light that was less than 100 feet from our campus when suddenly someone ran a red light and completely broadsided our car. This accident left me in a coma [unconscious] for over a month with traumatic brain injury. My life will forever be altered because of that.

The accident impaired my speech in a big way. I wasn't able to respond as quickly in conversations as most people do. My reaction time is slowly getting better, but at first it was awful. One of my biggest problems was with memory. When talking with friends, I would completely forget what the topic was and have to continually ask what was going on. I would forget words often, too, even the really simple ones. I could act out what I was trying to say, and people would have to guess. Once they said the word I was trying to say, I would remember it. As a result, I am much quieter than I was before.

Text isn't bad for me, but I struggle with it. It takes me much longer to read now. The accident caused me to be half-blind, so that also plays a big part in reading. My eyes scan the paper much slower than they used to. When I have a test in school, I am permitted to go in my own room and take as much time as I want. Teachers give me that option because I would not be able to take the test with other students without going way over the time allowed.

I sometimes overanalyze a person's body language and what it means. My opinion of how I read this is since my speech was heavily damaged by the accident, I have better perception of people's body language. I can tell their attitudes and their tone of voice better as well. After two years since the accident, I react faster and speak louder and faster. I am still making progress, slow but there.

I would tell others to just keep pushing. Progress depends upon outlook. There was a time when I thought I would never make it, that I'd be stuck where I was forever. Then one day some friends from college visited. They told me stories of what we used to do and funny things I said. I decided I wanted to be the "old Shannon" again. So I created a positive outlook on what was happening. And look where I am now—back to college, away from home, and maintaining above a 3.0 GPA![a]

The odd thing is how unpredictable and complex brain injury can be. According to the Brain Injury Association of America, no two brain injuries are exactly the same. Resulting disabilities from brain injury depend upon the cause, intensity of trauma, and where in the brain the blow hits. In a matter of seconds, brain injury "can change everything about us—who we are, and the way we think, act, and feel."[2]

About 1.7 million people in the United States experience traumatic brain damage each year.[3] Injury can result from any number of causes. They range from falls and physical assault to vehicle crashes, sporting accidents, and strokes. Falls account for 35 percent of all brain injury, but car crashes contribute 17 percent, other assaults cause 10 percent, and sports/recreational events cause more than 16 percent. You don't need to walk around being scared of every move you make, but you do need to stay alert to potentially dangerous situations.

How the Brain Works

Your brain is actually pretty soft, even though it comes encased in a hard protective skull. The soft core is made up of delicate nerve cells that form pathways throughout the brain, like roots in a plant. These pathways carry messages to various parts of the brain. Each part has a specific job and connects with other parts of the brain to coordinate more complex operations. In turn, portions of the brain send messages throughout the body to control your body systems. These systems direct you to perform different functions they control and monitor, such as heart rate, movement, and senses.

Besides specific parts, scientists divide the brain into main sections called *lobes*. Each lobe from front to back is the locus of specific body functions. For example, the frontal lobe that lies approximately inside your forehead monitors attention and concentration, emotions, problem solving, judgment, personality characteristics, and speaking. So any trauma to that area can bring changes to your entire functioning, especially in communication.

Your brain comes divided into right and left sides. Many researchers have conducted studies to determine what it means to be a dominant right brain or left brain person. Researchers claim the right side of the brain is the creative, big picture, imaginative side. The left brain tells you to be more logical, analytical, and organized. Usually, individuals are a combination of the two, but most have preferences and skills that remind them which side their brain favors.

How the Brain Works after Brain Trauma

When trauma strikes parts of the brain that control language, a disorder can occur. Even areas of the brain that deal with balance and muscle coordination contribute to problems moving the tongue or lips, which affect speaking. Brain injury to motor areas can cause slurring, slower rate of speech, harsh voice, or lowered volume. Injuries to the right side of our brain contribute to loss of creativity and music perception, visual memory, and control over left-side body movements.

Injuries to the left side of the brain may produce difficulty with body movements. On the right side, symptoms from injury center on logic, verbal memory, and speaking, expressing, or understanding language. With injuries to both sides, scattered damage can inhibit general thinking, speed of thought processes, attention, and concentration.[4]

Comparing brain injury to a broken bone, for example, illustrates how important it is to protect the brain and nervous system. According to ThinkFirst, a foundation devoted to educating people about how to make safer choices, the typical broken arm heals in between six to eight weeks. Although weakness may

Sabrina's Story

Eighteen-year-old Sabrina had a 10 percent chance of living after being hit on the head with a lead pipe. She doesn't remember the accident. But she remembers waking up in the hospital unable to speak, walk, or eat, even swallow. Every skill had to be relearned, and the journey was slow going.

Once Sabrina was home, her family was thrilled but scared for her. Her mom was overprotective, and Sabrina couldn't go out. Once Sabrina was able to walk and talk, she was better able to handle the remaining challenges. Gradually, her mom adjusted to having a daughter with learning differences.

At school Sabrina worried people would treat her differently, and they did. Many approached her like a two-year-old. When she started dating, boys thought she'd be a pushover because she wasn't as smart.

With time, Sabrina discovered ways to cope with the depression and desperation that followed. Most importantly, she decided to talk about her brain injury. She discovered that talking not only relieved her pent-up feelings, but it helped others understand what she was going through. Admitting she was different from brain injury allowed her to ask for what she needed or didn't understand.

Sabrina also learned that true friends supported her. As for dating, she realized she just needed to find the right person. She allowed herself to still have goals and want to continue her education. But she knew she'd have to take these goals one at a time.[b]

continue for a while, the arm will work as soon as a cast is removed. With movement, the arm starts building muscle again. But the brain's nerve tissues cannot heal the same way as skin and bones, meaning head trauma could result in permanent damage. ThinkFirst wants you to know that most traumas are preventable, if you know how to stay safe and make healthful choices (see the Resources section).

Adolescents and Brain Injury

Adolescents and young adults ages fifteen to twenty-four are at the highest risk for brain injury. This is probably because teens are more active and move about with less adult supervision, which is a good thing. Moreover, teens tend to become involved in more sporting activities. Adolescents in general have fewer fears that contribute to taking greater risks. The next most susceptible is the zero to four-year-old crowd, who tumble and jump without thinking. After the youngest population, injury hits seniors over age seventy-five years who lose their balance more frequently.

In all categories, males receive more blows to the head than females. Researchers believe that this is because males engage in riskier behaviors more often than females. But this doesn't leave females off the hook for sudden injury. Both males and females can wind up in situations that increase chances of TBI and resulting language disorders.

Recovering from Traumatic Brain Injury

If you or anyone you know feels a headache that won't quit or seems disoriented after being hit or jarred, the Brain Injury Association of America has some tips about what to do—or not do—to feel better and heal faster.[c]

1. First and foremost consult with a doctor, if you suspect head injury. This discomfort isn't something to deny.
2. Tell the doctor about any medications currently being taken. Only ingest what the doctor approves, as medicine can make matters worse for head injury. Similarly, never drink alcohol or ingest other mind-altering substances with head injury. They can magnify your symptoms or cause new ones.

3. Rest. Refrain from resuming normal activities, school, work, or chores, no matter how tempting. The game can go on without you. No game is worth permanent damage of any kind, especially to the head.

4. Stay away from activities that can put you in danger of another blow or head jarring. More blows mean bigger problems that can compound over time.

5. Wait until the doctor OK's operating moving vehicles or equipment, and that includes bicycles, skateboards, and cars.

6. Keep a diary or list of things you want to remember, if memory is affected. This includes information and reactions that are important to share with your doctor.

7. Work with a speech and language therapist familiar with brain injury, if the problem seems severe and/or involves communication. Individuals get better, even with terrible head injuries, after seeing the appropriate health-care professional.

Aphasia

A TBI may cause aphasia, a far-reaching language disorder that can strike anyone at any time. According to the Center for Neurobiology of Language Recovery headquartered at Northwestern University, aphasia alters the lives of more than 1 million people in the United States. About 80,000 new cases appear each year.[5]

In the chapter 5 opener, Oliver Sacks presents an amazing description of how some people with aphasia might react. Although he focuses on specific reactions to a speech, a range of symptoms may accompany aphasia. But what exactly is aphasia? What is involved with aphasia? How does someone acquire this strange communication disorder?

The word *aphasia* comes from a Greek word meaning "loss of speech." But rather than a total inability to speak, aphasia is categorized as a language disorder by modern speech pathologists. That is because of what occurs during the condition. Either incoming or outgoing messages can be affected. Therefore, aphasia contributes to problems understanding, reading, or writing in addition to trouble speaking.

"The interesting thing about aphasia is it doesn't affect any other cognitive systems," says Northwestern professor and aphasia expert Cynthia Thompson.

"These people are intelligent. They're not impaired, except for when they need to use language, either reading, writing, talking, or listening."[6]

Aphasia is a common result of brain injury. The brain controls a series of events required to speak and understand language. Any assault or resulting blockage to these events occurring can disrupt normal speech and language. Most often, the left side of the brain experiences the assault, as that is the part of the brain responsible for language.

Impaired language can appear after stroke, head injury, a brain tumor, or other worsening brain disease. Depending upon location of the brain injury and which parts are affected, aphasia can be expressive (ability to speak usable language) or receptive (ability to understand incoming language). If someone experiences both types of language impairment, their condition is called global aphasia.

Signs of Aphasia

Symptoms of aphasia can be mild or severe. They vary widely from person to person. In some cases, aphasia can be a fleeting problem lasting a few minutes, such as with a migraine headache. Many people with mild or moderate damage completely recover any lost language skills. But 1 in 300 people with more extreme forms of brain damage may suffer lasting aphasia to a greater or lesser degree.

At the mildest levels, aphasia contributes to difficulty with finding the right word or using the wrong word in place of what someone wants to say. Words most affected are nouns, especially proper names. You might notice problems you or your parents have remembering names with age. These infrequent lapses are usually not aphasia, just part of the normal aging process.

Kristen's Story

Kristen explained her journey with aphasia to therapists at Northwestern's Aphasia and Neurolinguistics Research Laboratory. It began when she experienced a stroke at age thirty-one. She was working as a physical therapist and engaged to be married. Suddenly, everything disappeared. She couldn't talk at all for two weeks. When she uttered her first word, it was "guacamole." Kristen entered a language therapy program. For the next three years, she met with therapists twice a week. Slowly, she regained the ability to speak. But five years later, she still speaks in short, planned sentences.[d]

People with more severe levels of expressive aphasia might not be able to speak at all. If they do, they may sound slurred or garbled, like someone who just woke up or drank too much alcohol. They may be unable to read and write. Grammar rules go out the window, as people with expressive aphasia struggle to complete sentences and thoughts. Or they may find it difficult to understand what others are saying.

In his book *The Mind's Eye*, Oliver Sacks talks about aphasia patients who could only utter single words like "Damn!" or "Fine!" One woman only said, "Thank you, Mama" after her stroke.[7] Even when experiencing these or similar problems, however, people with aphasia usually continue to think clearly. This disconnect between thoughts and speaking or writing can be frustrating to anyone with aphasia—and those around them.

Although aphasia strikes at any age, more people acquire the condition in their middle or older years. This is one language disorder that affects males and females equally. The National Institutes of Health estimate that about 80,000 people become aphasic each year. Currently, about 1 million individuals live with aphasia,[8] but numbers will probably climb as the population of older Americans continues to rise.

Identifying Aphasia

Most often, anyone with brain injury first receives care in the hospital from a neurologist, a doctor who treats conditions of the nervous system, which includes the brain. Once the trauma becomes stable but a communication problem lingers, the neurologist will probably recommend a complete evaluation from a speech and language pathologist. The evaluation usually covers tests of speaking, comprehending, reading, and writing.

Causes of Brain Injury: Stroke

With a stroke, assault to the brain comes from the inside, rather than a TBI from a collision or fall. Either a blood clot obstructs an artery or blood vessel, or the blood vessel leaks or bursts. Each case disrupts the flow of blood to areas of the brain that influence language. Without blood supplying oxygen to speech and language centers, brain cells die within a few minutes or hours, interfering with communication.

Strokes are the third-leading cause of death in the United States, and they are more common in older people. Risk of stroke doubles each decade after age fifty-five. But that picture may be changing. Two risk factors can appear at any age. One is a blood vessel or artery weakness or defect from birth that can rear

What Can Therapy Do for Aphasia?

The National Institutes of Health currently funds the Center for the Neurobiology of Language Recovery. The program, headquartered at Northwestern University in Illinois, coordinates research from Johns Hopkins, Harvard, and Boston universities. College researchers are using brain imaging techniques to investigate language recovery when blood flow resumes after stroke and other brain trauma. They hope to collect information that will predict how well and under which circumstances language can best return.[e]

In some cases, a person with aphasia may recover without any treatment. But most aphasia patients will need some form of therapy. No matter what age, someone with aphasia can benefit from speech therapy. Therapists work on helping clients express thoughts or understand what is heard or read. They empower clients by teaching strategies for different communication situations. They work with family members and friends to suggest ways to make communication easier. And they give patients and their families hope and support for each step on the sometimes rough path toward improvement.

Therapists can also suggest communication aids, such as hearing aids, glasses, magnifying aids, pictures, and other technology, writing, and amplification devices that will stimulate language. They recommend ways to enhance communication interactions. Some suggestions include

- giving plenty of time for responses;
- asking questions to make sure someone with aphasia understands, using short, simple sentences for requests or exchanging information;
- encouraging other forms of communication, such as gestures or drawing; and
- keeping environments free of distractions, such as a loud radio or television that may interfere with clear communication.

Most of all, a therapist can remind loved ones that the person with aphasia still has intelligence, common sense, and a sense of humor. If you know someone with aphasia, you need to remember to cherish and try to bring out these qualities.

Senator Mark Kirk Returns to Washington after a Stroke

There were no Democrats or Republicans lining the U.S. Capitol steps when Republican senator Mark Kirk began his climb toward work. Only well-wishers gathered to support his comeback to Congress after a long absence. What mattered was the fact that he was back.

Kirk had recently spent several months in intense therapy to improve how he moved and talked after a stroke. Seven months earlier, the fifty-two-year-old senator had experienced a terrible headache and numbness. His doctor ordered him to the hospital immediately. At the hospital, Kirk's doctor confirmed that a blood clot had developed from an artery tear in his neck. The clot dislodged and traveled to the right side of his brain, causing dangerous swelling and lack of feeling in the left side of his body.

Luckily, Kirk lived, and the trauma was on the right side of the brain. His ability to think remained intact. But his motor skills suffered the greatest damage, with lasting impairment to the left side of his body. The assault in the motor areas also interfered with the rhythm and flow of his speech.

Once doctors stabilized Kirk, the long days of therapy began. He had speech therapy. He practiced walking on his feet with a harness and holding onto side rails to prevent falling. He became pen pal with eleven-year-old Jackson Cunningham, also partly paralyzed from a stroke, who encouraged Kirk on his long journey to recovery.

Cunningham wrote Kirk early on, "Here's some advice. Do not give up on yourself."[f]

Kirk determined to return to the Senate, even if that meant in a wheelchair. But that first day back, he climbed the forty-five stairs to the capitol door by foot. He had help from others, but the drive to succeed was all his doing. Today, he still works to speak more fluently, and he tires easily. But, like his inspiration Jackson Cunningham, Kirk inspires others with his drive to be a role model and a productive senator.

its ugly head at any time. The other involves the increase in young people who have type 1 or type 2 diabetes. These two conditions affect large and small blood vessels. Type 1 diabetes cannot be prevented. But type 2 can usually be avoided by keeping weight in check and limiting sugary snacks.

Causes of Brain Injury: Aggression/Gun Assaults

About 10 percent of individuals with brain injury sustain their trauma from unwanted assault. Numbers for nonmilitary gun violence, in particular, are staggering. Totals are second only to automobile crashes as the cause of brain injury deaths in the United States. And this doesn't count the many soldiers returning from active duty where they survived debilitating bombings. According to the National Center for Injury Prevention and Control, the leading cause of death for ages eight through nineteen years is firearms. In 2010 alone, 2,433 teens died from firearm violence, including 749 who used guns to kill themselves by suicide.

Even when gun violence is nonfatal, the risks remain high for TBIs for the 15,428 who survive. More than 11,929 live after a gun attack, 254 outlive a suicide attempt, and 3,164 survive an accidental shooting. Many live with language disorders triggered after gun trauma to the brain. With statistics like these, many groups seek to limit the number of available guns and create rules to keep them from the hands of potentially violent teens and adults.

Gun owners can reduce TBIs from firearms by hiding them unloaded in a securely locked place. They should keep ammunition separate from the guns, and never let kids and teens get the idea that guns are for playing with. You may think guns are a power trip, but they're not. They are weapons that harm or kill!

As for reducing suicides, teens can reduce thoughts of death by seeking out a trusted adult to talk about feeling sad or depressed. If you know someone who is thinking about suicide, direct him or her to a trusted adult or one of the websites in the Resources section. Depressed teens who attempt suicide use guns more than any other method. Teens at risk for suicide often have made prior suicide attempts, have a family history of suicide, abuse drugs, or have experienced abuse or trauma. They need help!

Similarly, you need to hang around adult role models who resolve fights and arguments nonviolently and without guns. If you have a say in your family, suggest to your parents that the best way to reduce risk of gun accidents is to remove them from the home completely, particularly if you have younger brothers and sisters. Kids are naturally curious, no matter what parents say.

On the government level, you and your friends can be proactive about gun safety. Contact local officials to enact laws to change this nation's gun culture. Show support for a more peaceful community by working to enact laws that limit assault weapons and the number of rounds for other types of guns. Encourage lawmakers to tackle requirements for universal background checks for all gun owners and to close loopholes that allow less strict rules for sales at gun shows than at stores. Moreover, let media producers and their advertisers know you prefer more family-friendly shows on television and in movies that don't involve solving problems with guns.

Guns Never Silenced Congresswoman Giffords

On January 8, 2011, Arizona congresswoman Gabby Giffords approached a waiting crowd in a grocery store parking lot. As she began to speak, a lone gunman opened fire. He first hit Giffords in the back of the head, then killed six people and wounded another thirteen with a volley of thirty-three rounds.

Miraculously, the congresswoman survived, but her life since has forever changed. Giffords was shot at close range in the back of the head in the brain's left hemisphere. The injury left her right side paralyzed, altering how she uses her hands and walks. Her language recall, expression, and fluency took a huge hit, making speaking difficult and frustrating. She knows what she wants to convey but often cannot.

Giffords received intense speech therapy that included music therapy. News coverage showed a lively Giffords singing what she wanted to say. Speech therapists know that when motor areas of the brain remain intact, as with Giffords, the patient can bypass problems by singing instead of talking. Now Giffords uses her left hand to navigate her iPad. She still has difficulty with fluency, talking in partial or choppy sentences. She also has challenges calling up words she wants to express.

But Giffords will not be silenced. She constantly remembers the thirteen-year-old girl and others who lost their lives that day because they wanted to learn more about her and their government. Giffords may never return to Congress, but she and her husband, Mark Kelly, speak out to improve gun laws, so others won't have to experience what their family has. They started Americans for Responsible Solutions (see Resources), a group that raises money to counter the National Rifle Association lobbying to limit gun control laws. Giffords stands in the center of the debate to expand background checks for gun buyers at gun shows and reduce rounds available for a given gun. Only now when time and words count most, her husband makes the important calls to press lawmakers for greater gun controls.

Causes of Brain Injury: Auto and Motorcycle Crashes

There is a reason states have increased ages for teens who want a driver's license. Many districts enacted rules to extend driver's education and time spent as a driver-in-training with a responsible adult. These requirements are a response to the fact that individuals between ages fifteen and twenty-four years represent 14 percent of the U.S. population. Yet, this age group accounts for 29 percent of motor vehicle injuries. In 2010, 2,700 teens between ages sixteen and nineteen died, and 282,000 were treated in emergency rooms for vehicle crashes.[9] That adds up to a lot of TBI and increased problems with language disorders. In fact, motor crashes are a leading cause of brain injuries among the fifteen-to-twenty-year-old set.

Several factors contribute to high rates of car accidents. One is the teen makeup. Adolescents are more adventurous and think less of consequences. It's true: brain imaging studies display these reactions. So teens are more likely than older drivers to speed. They leave shorter distances between their vehicle and the one in front. And they neglect signs of danger that would ensure they and their passengers wear seat belts and stay attentive to the road. Beyond the teen driver's natural psyche, more risk comes from having another teen, especially a male, in the same car.[10]

Another problem is teenage drinking. Research shows that fewer teens drive drunk than a decade or two ago, which is great. Still, teens are more likely to drive all sorts of vehicles, including motorcycles, drunk than drivers from other age groups. About half the car crashes arise from drug or alcohol use. Additionally, more accidents occur between midnight and 3 a.m. and on weekends, although as Shannon noted, traffic crashes can happen any time of day when someone isn't paying attention.

Drug use among teens continues to cause problems with driving—and other issues that extend later in life. About 50 percent of brain injury due to car crashes results from drug or alcohol use. According to the Brain Injury Association of America and other medical sources, drugs affect teens' developing brains more than brains of older folks. Marijuana studies show that smoking alters hearing, coordination, and perceptions of all kinds and blocks messages entering the brain. Any drug fogs thinking and slows reaction time. You can imagine what these problems do to driving safely.

Over time, the brain becomes injured from drugs in many ways, including memory and ability to socialize. Since drugs like marijuana are often illegal, except in states where medical marijuana is monitored for purity, teens have no way to know if the drugs they might buy are pure. It's not like they can ask a professional who knows. Any chemicals to enhance addiction can be added by underworld and shady sellers. All drugs increase the risk of injury behind the wheel.

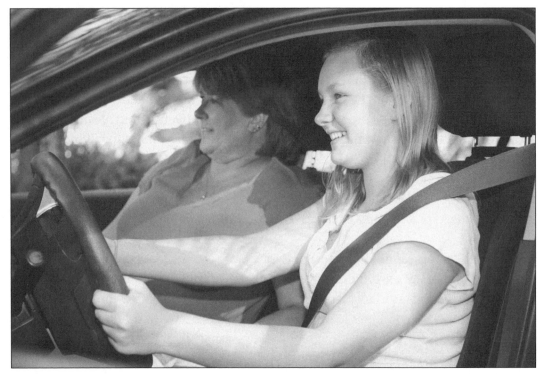

Teen drives with a parent or instructor until she feels confident enough to travel solo.

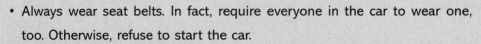

Driving Habits That Reduce the Risk of TBI

Here are some suggestions for preventing driving accidents:

- Always wear seat belts. In fact, require everyone in the car to wear one, too. Otherwise, refuse to start the car.
- Obey speed limits. That's one way to keep control of the car. Drive slower when road conditions are slippery or otherwise dangerous.
- Designate a driver, if you go somewhere where there is drinking or drugs or both. Don't assume you or a friend who drinks are fine to drive. Never go in a car driven by someone who has ingested alcohol or drugs. Studies show that even the smallest alcohol level can impair driving enough to cause an accident. If no one is fit to drive, either call a responsible adult

or friend or stay put. You can drive home alone or with others once you have slept off whatever it is you ingested at the party. Of course, the best idea is to not drink or get high at all.

- Be an alert and careful pedestrian. Even being a drunk or stoned pedestrian can prove dangerous. Drugs not only impair judgment and reaction time, they can cause paranoia and hallucinations that play havoc with approaching headlights and the ability to judge distances.

- Don't let someone else who has been drinking or taking drugs walk anywhere, especially alone. Impaired judgment puts someone in danger, even when crossing the street. Either call a cab, find a responsible escort, or as with driving, encourage the person to stay put until sober.

- New drivers should drive solo for several months after receiving a license. Research shows that passengers increase the crash risk of untested drivers. Passengers, eating and drinking, and arranging hair or applying cosmetics while driving all distract from the main goal—to drive somewhere safely. These tips work for experienced drivers, too.

- Never text while driving. And don't talk on cell phones or block out sounds with earbuds. Drivers need to stay alert—to the road and to horns that warn them of danger.

- Refrain from multitasking. No matter how adept you might be at accomplishing several tasks at once, this mode of operating doesn't mix with driving. Studies prove that individuals are not as good as they think at multitasking. If you absolutely must respond to a text or call a friend, pull over until you finish the conversation. You don't want to wind up kissing a tree because you took your eyes off the road for a split second, which is all an accident takes to occur.

- Work with your parents or guardians on a graduated approach to driving, even if your state/community does not require a slow entry into driving. Drive with a responsible adult until you both feel comfortable with you driving solo.

- Know rules of the road and laws in your community, and review them regularly. Your safe journey depends upon obeying driving rules.

Causes of Brain Injury: Roller Sports

Roller sports—inline skates, skateboards, bicycles, and scooters—can be great fun to operate. Until they produce injuries. One report noted that nearly half of all kid head injuries in 2000 came from a combination of bicycling, skating, and skateboarding. Of emergency room visits, cycling caused 56 percent of the problems. But more than 100,000 inline and 50,000 skateboarding injuries extreme enough to warrant emergency room care occur each year. The report further noted that 90 percent of these injuries could have been prevented.[11]

You might think the fall is so short a distance that nothing serious can happen. But TBI can result from falls of as little a two feet above ground. ThinkFirst, the national brain injury prevention organization, believes 85 percent of all scooter and inline skating injuries can be prevented by wearing a proper helmet and other safety gear.[12]

What should a teen do? First, always wear protective headgear. Make sure the helmet at least meets safety standards developed by the American Society for Testing and Materials. Remember that skateboard and bicycle helmets offer different protections, so buy the one that matches the sport. Next, make sure to follow safe guidelines. Stay on smooth surfaces, and skate during daylight. As with other wheeled vehicles, obey traffic rules. Experienced rollers say to stay off streets, never hitch a ride from bicycles or cars, and only use one skateboard per person, no matter how much fun and enticing doubling seems.

For skating, prevention involves warming up by practicing braking and stopping before starting on a longer excursion. Once on a path, be courteous and pass on the left. Announce intentions to those already on the sidewalk. Check the skateboard regularly for cracks or other damage, which should be a regular activity before using a scooter, too.

Everett's Story

High school sophomore Everett Zamarron-Smith wasn't wearing a helmet when his skateboard sped out of control on a steep street. Life changed for him and his family the moment his head slammed on the concrete. Everett now had to work on therapy for memory loss, motor loss throughout his body, and trouble communicating. Meanwhile, his mother, Delva, had to leave her job to tend to a six-foot-one son who was helpless as a baby. But she forces herself and her son to be positive. She advocates for helmet use and boosts her son's morale, telling him how far he's come with talking and walking. When Everett hears the positive message, he grins and lifts his fist saying "Yea!"[9]

Safe Tips for Bicycles and Motorcycles

Bicycles and motorcycles can risk health and safety as much as a car and result in an accident and TBI. Here are guidelines that might prevent disastrous consequences:

- Wear a helmet, and make sure it's one that fits snug enough to stay on your head, if you fall. In some states, helmets are the law. With all others, it's just a smart prevention measure.
- The same suggestions apply about driving impaired, whether with alcohol or drugs. Don't risk being on the road when your mind is elsewhere.
- Know and follow local laws. That includes knowing hand turning gestures and where to ride on the road.
- Be practical and stay alert. Riding to the right side of the road works—unless someone exits a parked car. Watch that driveways and parking lots are free of moving cars, or people for that matter.
- Buy a headlight and rear light or reflector for night riding.
- Wear a reflective vest or safety triangle to make sure you are visible at sundown, sunup, or nighttime when light is reduced.
- Invest in a horn or bell that is loud enough to warn passing cars and pedestrians where you are.
- Slow down at corners, crosswalks, or near pedestrians. Remember that young children, animals, and older folks can be unpredictable and/or not pay attention to approaching bicycles or motorcycles. Loud motorcycles can flummox some pedestrians, too. Be prepared to stop, or go around spooked people or animals quickly.
- Attach a rearview mirror to your bicycle and motorcycle to increase visibility.
- Avoid busy and narrow streets for riding.
- Leave the iPod or other music device at home. You need to be able to focus on traffic instead of music.
- Check out this website for other bicycle safety ideas: Michael Bluejay, "Bicycle Safety: How to Not Get Hit by Cars," BicycleSafe.com.

Causes of Brain Injury: Water Play

Swimming, water sports, and boating provide loads of fun, too. But they also contribute to large numbers of teens exposed to acquiring brain damage, that is, if you don't follow safety rules in the water. Doctors say it takes only two minutes to lose consciousness and four to six minutes to wind up with permanent brain damage from either being submerged underwater too long or hitting your head after a shallow dive. Not good for your communication skills and leading a normal life. And not a good trade-off for an hour or two of fun without taking precautions.

Here are some recommendations for making the next water experience a fun, yet safe, one:

- If you dive, know the water and ground conditions before leaping. Enter water with feet first to test how deep it gets, how quickly, and what type of landing the section of water provides. Many diving accidents occur in natural bodies of water that are unstable and dangerous. Above-ground pools are not made for diving. And never dive when water is less than nine feet deep. Ninety percent of diving injuries come after dives in less than six feet of water.
- When swimming, bring a buddy along. If you prefer solitary swims, at least make sure you are in shouting range of other people. Of course, swimming within earshot of a lifeguard is the safest situation.
- Be alert to undercurrents, undertows, and changing waves. Swimming near a lifeguard will ensure you gain this type of information beforehand and can gauge your swim accordingly. Sometimes, you may encounter surprises, or you may misjudge distances and swim farther away from shore than intended and experience problems. If caught in an undertow that's sweeping you away from shore, swim parallel to the shoreline until you can break from the rip current. Then swim back to shore safely.
- When boating, you need to wear Coast Guard–approved life jackets and know rules of the water where you are sailing or motoring.
- Two preventive measures that apply to all water activities are (1) never participate after drinking or taking drugs and (2) learn CPR. You never know when the latter skill will come in handy.

Causes of Brain Injury: Team Sports

Sports and recreational activities give rise to a large share of teen brain injuries. Many are extensive enough to alter language development. These injuries can

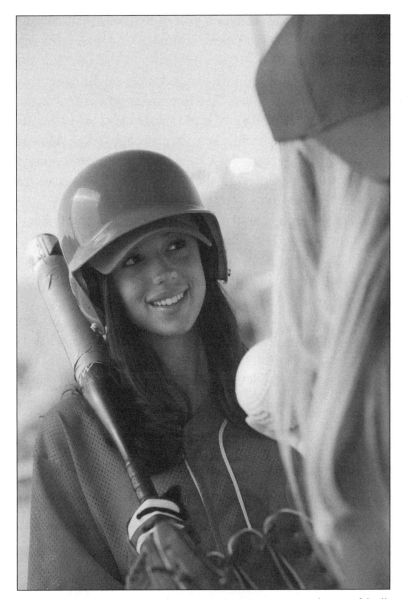

Coaches are discovering that more team sports, such as softball, require proper protective gear.

cause behavior and language problems that affect school and relationships. In the past, coaches and team members believed that if teens got hurt, well, they should suck it up and continue playing. Thankfully, that mentality is starting to change.

The difference in attitude is based on recent reports that support how delicate the developing teen brain is. Dr. Jonathon Fellius from the Kessler Institute of Traumatic Brain Injury believes that "the brain is a delicate jellyfish matrix, vulnerable to sudden physical blows, . . . despite the thick case of bone that surrounds it." He knows that the adolescent brain is not fully developed until you reach at least twenty-five years of age. Some injuries are so subtle they go unnoticed until one final blow causes a severe reaction that cannot be ignored. Fellius stresses that even in cases where scans look normal after injury, damage could be occurring.[13]

Studies show that blows are cumulative, meaning slight damage develops into bigger problems with each new blow. So a few small blows can eventually produce huge life-changing alterations in how someone behaves and functions. Another study on rats discovered that brain chemistry changes after damage from TBI. Several athletes have told reporters how they lost memory and other skills as they aged, even after they stopped playing their sport. And there have been links between TBI and suicide attempts.

With 60 percent of high school students and growing numbers of preteens participating in team sports, handling concussions and other brain injuries is a major public health concern. According to the National Football League, football alone results in brain injuries in 1 of every 3.5 games.[14] And 3.5 million kids between ages six and thirteen play football in the United States.

In reaction to recent news, the National Football League, colleges, and high school teams have changed how athletes practice. Once coaches believed that players needed to be hit and hit hard during practice to prepare them for game force from other teams. Now all levels bar spear tackling, when one player tackles another headfirst.

Headache of a Story

When Marlee was in junior high, she went ice skating with friends at the local rink. Never much of an athlete, she stayed in the corner and away from faster skaters. But the corner wasn't enough to keep her safe. While practicing skating backward, Marlee slid onto her bottom. She was padded enough when she landed, but her head flung backward, cracking on the ice. She wound up dazed and off balance enough to stop skating. Since she was embarrassed about her lack of skating skills, she never told anyone about the head-bashing fall. After a few days her headache went away.

Fast forward a few years. Marlee was getting into a cab but didn't clear the top of the doorway. The result was enough of a blow to cause a headache that lasted for more than two weeks. Since she was leaving town, she never thought to get her head examined. But between the two blows, Marlee wonders if they contribute to her having more problems calling up words than friends her age experience.[h]

Coaches have also reduced the amount of contact drills during practice. One national youth organization of hundreds of thousands of football teams, Pop Warner, enacted new rules that limited contact drills to no more than one-third of practice. Another group, USA Football, has begun a Safe Tackling program to teach coaches and players in independent football leagues how to tackle safely.[15]

The National Football League decided their professional players cost too much to have their careers cut short by a bang to the head. Nowadays, training camps follow a new practice model. Most tackling is prohibited. Only minimal contact between players is tolerated, and that occurs no more than five minutes a week. Mostly, players practice a form of touch football. Other fights and forceful shoves are quickly broken up as well. As New York Giants' coach Tom Coughlin said after he interrupted a brawl between two players, "There's no place for that. Somebody could get hurt."[16]

These actions reflect new state laws about how to handle concussions from sports. *Concussion* is the term used for a form of TBI from a jolt or blow that is hard enough to alter the way the brain usually works. In 2009, Washington State

Know When to Stop Playing Due to Concussion

Anyone who likes to play sports needs to be aware of possible concussion. Whenever a blow to the head or body jerks you enough to cause your head to jolt quickly, you may be in line for a concussion. But how do you know if one happens?

Any time you hit your head and later feel a headache or pressure that won't quit or feel like you want to vomit, these might be signs of concussion. Also, be alert to sound and light sensitivity, double or blurry vision, dizziness or balance issues, or feeling sluggish, confused, or down and unable to concentrate or remember things. These are signs to sit out the game and head for a doctor. And be sure to allow someone to escort you, rather than go it alone.

Even if your coach insists you are fine to play, trust your judgment and stand your ground. If you wind up without a concussion, your brain still has undergone a trauma and needs a long time to rest before playing again. If you find you do have a concussion, give yourself time to feel better, no matter how frustrating a slow recovery or enticing joining other activities can be.

became the first to pass a concussion-in-sports law. The next month, Oregon passed its own. By 2012, forty-three states had enacted laws, often called return-to-play laws, that produced guidelines for contact practice. Guidelines ensure that sports equipment remains in working order; information is posted for parents, coaches, and athletes at schools and on the field; and data is collected to improve safety during sports. Many guidelines go even further, directing schools how to handle students who suffer a concussion.

Although football and ice hockey, two contact sports, lead the pack in sports-related brain injuries, other sports take their toll, too. Consider that 10 percent of all college and 20 percent of high school athletes experience a concussion during any single season. The federal government reports scary statistics of concussions from various contact sports. From a 2007 report, tallies indicated that about 25 percent of sports injuries came from winter sports, such as ice hockey, skiing, and sledding. And 11.7 percent of teens who ride horses sustain concussions from horseback riding. Although these sports can produce a concussion, most can be avoided by playing safely.

Resources

Organizations

Americans for Responsible Solutions
P.O. Box 15642
Washington, DC 20003
www.americansforresponsiblesolutions.org
Organization started by former congresswoman Gabby Giffords and her husband, Mark Kelly, after she and several others were shot. The group seeks reasonable criminal background checks, limits on high-capacity guns and the ability to buy assault weapons, and an end to gun trafficking.

Brady Campaign
1225 Eye Street NW, Suite 1100
Washington, DC 20005
202-898-0792
www.bradycampaign.org
Organization to prevent gun violence that was started by Sarah Brady and her husband Jim, former press secretary to President Ronald Reagan, who suffered partial paralysis and brain injury after an attempt to kill the president. The group seeks to keep guns from criminals and the mentally ill and to promote gun safety for the 300 million guns in U.S. communities.

Brain Injury Association of America
1608 Spring Hill Road, Suite 110
Vienna, VA 22182
703-761-0750
800-444-6443 (hotline)
www.biausa.org
Resource organization for information about brain injury and host of the National
Brain Injury Information Center.

National Aphasia Association
350 Seventh Avenue, Suite 902
New York, NY 10001
800-922-4622
www.aphasia.org
Organization that offers public education, research, and support services to people with aphasia and their families.

National Highway Traffic Safety Administration
1200 N. Jersey Avenue SE, West Building
Washington, DC 20590
888-327-4236
www.nhtsa.gov
Federal organization that handles vehicle safety and has a web page called "Bicycling" with safety tips.

National Information on Disabilities and Communication Disorders Information
Clearinghouse
1 Communication Avenue
Bethesda, MD 20892-3456
800-241-1044
www.nidcd.nih.gov
National resource for communication and aphasia information, such as www
.nidcd.nih.gov/health/voice/pages/aphasia.aspx.

Safe Kids Worldwide/National Safe Kids Campaign
1301 Pennsylvania Avenue NW, Suite 1000
Washington, DC 20004
202-662-0600
www.safekids.org
Worldwide nonprofit organization and campaign to prevent injuries in kids and
teens through education and resources that was founded by Dr. Martin Eichelberger

of Children's National Medical Center in Washington, DC and funded by Johnson & Johnson.

ThinkFirst National Injury Prevention Foundation
1801 N. Mill Street, Suite F
Naperville, IL 60563
630-393-1400
www.thinkfirst.org
National organization formed by frustrated neurologists who wanted to spread the word that young people don't have to experience serious injuries, if they can think first and prevent traumas from happening. The group focuses on a comprehensive education that includes school presentations and resource information about teens making safe choices that will reduce emergency room visits.

WHEN ENGLISH IS NEW OR SOUNDS DIFFERENT

Is it a disability when you need to learn another language so you can communicate where you live now? Do you have a disorder if you say letters and words differently from someone in another part of the country? How much of a problem is it if you learned English elsewhere, for example, India or Kenya, but need to be understood in the United States? Answers to these questions reside in whether what you say and how you say it interferes with learning at school, relating to friends, and interviewing for or understanding directions on the job. If the answer to these questions is yes, then perhaps you should request an evaluation and possibly assistance with tweaking your speech and language skills.

Bilingual Learners

Teens who are fluent in two languages are called bilingual. The National Center for Education Statistics claims that more than one in five school-aged children, or 21 percent, speak a language besides English at home. The center projects that number will climb as the immigrant population arriving in the United States increases.[1]

The United Nations Educational, Scientific and Cultural Organization estimates that about 6,800 languages are spoken throughout its international body of 195 member countries and eight associate members.[2] As the world shrinks with ever-new technology, more people from distant lands will either come to the United States or communicate with Americans through the Internet. Many more bilingual, even multilingual, children will be attending your schools. Hanging out with these classmates can be a great way to learn new languages, too.

Knowing more than one language is an advantage. You can talk with more people. You can communicate when you visit other countries. Research shows that knowing more than one language gives individuals a leg up with learning new words, listening, spelling, categorizing words, problem solving, and connecting with others.[3] These are all huge bonuses in the communication world!

In many parts of the world, children speak several languages before attending school. Papua New Guinea, an island nation in the South Pacific, has 5.8 million people, about the size of the Atlanta, Georgia, metropolitan area. Yet, the Papua speak about 715 languages across the country. That translates to every child learning several languages. A child grows up speaking one native language at home, another at the market, and possibly another at school. If students continue schooling, they usually learn in English. In fact, worldwide most education beyond high school is taught in English, a gift for Americans who know only their own language. But in the coming years, Americans can expect a greater need to learn more than one language in the United States.

Myths about Acquiring English

Studies show that bilingual students learn and develop speech and language skills in the same pattern as any other person their age. In fact, the idea that nonnatives do not want to learn and speak English is false. According to the PBS show *In the Mix* about teen immigrants from across the United States, there are not enough classes that teach English as a second language to meet the demand.

The other idea that nonnatives do not value education is far from the truth, too. Immigrants receive college degrees at the same 20 percent rate as English-speaking natives. And immigrants are twice as likely to earn more advanced degrees beyond four years of college.[4]

These statistics reinforce that any speech and language problems are not the result of knowing and speaking a second language. Chances are, if you experience difficulties learning in one language, these problems will occur no matter which language you speak and no matter how many you learn. If you learn languages easily, this, too, will cross language boundaries.

Being a Newcomer Isn't Easy Communication-wise

At times, bilingual students find that one language comes easier than the other. When you know one language better, the favored language is called the *dominant language*. This is the language you prefer to use for learning and socializing, if you have a choice. But to stay bilingual, you need to practice both languages on a regular basis. Otherwise, your nondominant language may fade with time. For example, you will probably forget the Spanish you learn in a high school class if you have no chance to use it.

Neema's Story

In 2013 PBS hosted a show called *In the Mix* to highlight the struggles of teens coming to America. One of the most compelling stories was from seventeen-year-old Neema. Two years before, she had arrived in the United States from Kenya, East Africa. She dreamed of what a wonderful country her new home would be. Although she spoke English in addition to Swahili, when she started high school she faced racism. Kids called her dumb because she was African. They said she should go back to Kenya—just because she had an accent. Neema was shocked because these people didn't know her. She believes people are not born racist. That comes from their surroundings.

As an immigrant Neema had to learn to respect other people's differences. She kept away from those who were negative toward her, or anyone, from somewhere else. She knows the school system where she lives is good. She sees how independent teens are there. Neema tries to make school better by valuing diversity. She helped start a diversity club at school. The club works to embrace differences. Someone told her, "If you were to turn us all inside out, wouldn't we look the same?"[a]

Many people who are not already fluent in two languages discover that learning a new language comes easily. For anyone who has an underlying speech and language problem, however, learning a new language can be stressful. Studies show that adopting a new language can take up to three years before someone develops enough language skill to feel comfortable talking socially, such as on the playground, in sports, or in discussing what's hot. Students may need four to seven years of formal instruction to develop enough language facility to easily understand schoolwork and take tests.

Even if students from another land seem fine talking socially, they may still bomb on tests. Not because they are dumb. They just haven't reached that level of language development needed to ace exams.

Other problems arise when teens are not solid in their native language. Perhaps they are behind in school or lacking strong grammar skills. Research confirms that success in school depends on learning concepts taught in a familiar language. If someone cannot grasp a skill in the first language, chances are it will not be clearer in the second language. These issues make it more difficult to succeed academically in an adopted land. The best predictor of academic success in

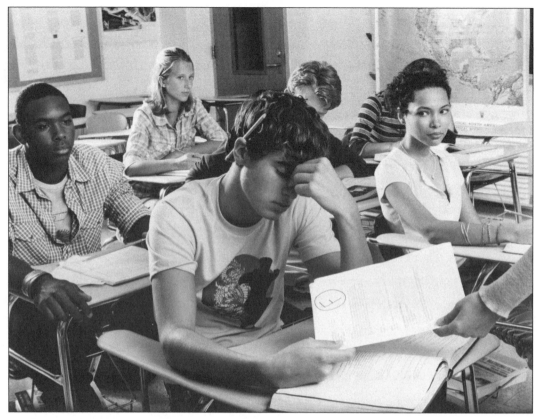

Student receives a low grade due to poor English language skills.

a new country is being capable of learning in the native language. Once a concept makes sense, then it easily transfers to another language.

For everyone, learning language vocabulary is key. Grammar and structure will come with time, but newcomers to the United States first need to expand the number of words they understand. Without a range of words, English language learners will be lost—in class or socializing with other students. People who have good language skills can transfer language word for word, such as learning the English word *pet* instead of the Spanish *mascota*. When a language other than English is spoken at home, newcomers have little exposure to English words. For many, going to school and making friends with English-speaking classmates outside their homes provides the only opportunities to hear and practice English.

The biggest disadvantage for someone new to English is how difficult the language is to learn. In Spanish, for example, most words are spelled the way they sound. For example with *zapato* (shoe), each letter is pronounced. In English there are dipthongs (two vowels in the same syllable saying one sound, such as the *oa* in *boat*), consonant blends (two consonants in the same syllable saying one sound, such as *th* in *thong*), two words spelled differently with different meanings but sounding the same (such as *bear* and *bare*), and a huge number of rules that make little sense to someone familiar with other grammar standards.

Be Kind to Those Who Speak Differently

Everyone wants the feeling of belonging. That may be more difficult if someone arrives from another country and is plopped into a strange land. Communities in the United States may have a different culture with different standards, rules, and language. As an American you want to—or should—be welcoming. One way is to reach out.

Here are some ideas for interacting with someone new to your class or neighborhood, someone who might speak another language, wear unusual clothes, and act differently. Many of these suggestions may seem obvious. But hey, everyone can use a little reminding once in a while.

- Never make fun of how someone speaks, acts, or dresses—and that includes allowing friends to do the same thing. Mimicking an accent: not cool. This includes making fun of accents from families that move from different parts of the United States, say from Charleston, South Carolina, to Boston, Massachusetts. This is "Do unto others as you would have them do unto you" territory.

- Try to picture yourself in their shoes. What would make you feel comfortable? What type of information would be helpful to learn about your new school, job, and community? Once you've done some self-examination, you can go about helping someone who you just met to adjust.

- Ask teens to talk about their country as a conversation starter. What do they like or miss about their former land? Ask what it's like to be a teen in that country. Identifying commonalities and differences is a good way to begin a relationship—and one of mutual understanding.

- Discuss what someone is expecting from this country. You can talk about what is realistic or not.

- Invite a newcomer to go places with you and your friends. Bowl together or attend sporting events or movies, eat at restaurants, or hang out at the mall. These are places that may be foreign to someone from elsewhere. Newcomers can expand their language as well as learn local traditions by going along.

- Watch television or visit popular Internet sites together. Share your younger siblings superhero apps that teach concept words, like *over*, *under*, and other basic direction words. These and similar apps are interesting for any age player and help build language.

- Suggest taking computer-aided language programs out of the library to work through together. These usually have pictures of beginning words, common phrases, and voice responses to hear how the words sound, which helps with practicing pronunciation.

- Remember that teens new to your country are not dumb for being unable to respond in class or answer your questions. Rather, they probably know too little English to feel comfortable speaking. They may be scared or feel uncomfortable. They may have experienced terrible horrors in their country of origin and be unsure of how others will react in their adopted country. Try to think of how you would feel living elsewhere, and act accordingly.

- Suggest checking out books on CD from the library. Reading along with the words helps with recognizing and pronouncing words in addition to re-inforcing vocabulary meaning. Another option is to read books for younger readers together. A preteen or teen may feel embarrassed to read "baby" books in front of classmates. But a true friend wouldn't tease friends who are trying to improve their language skills. Pick out common words in your language and the other person's. Look for root words (understand) and beginnings (*mis*understand) and endings (misunderstand*ing*) of words that would help someone pick out words and meanings.

Luincy's Story

Eight years ago, now seventeen-year-old Luincy came to the United States from the Dominican Republic. He remembers the first time he went to school was scary. His biggest struggle was language. Luincy felt terrible that he couldn't communicate with other people, so he didn't talk at all. He just listened, even though he couldn't figure out a word of what was being said. He says he felt so small and like the world was so big.[b]

Even when someone learns English rules, there are so many exceptions that English becomes awfully confusing. At least languages with pictograms, such as Chinese and Japanese, remain consistent once this type of alphabet is learned. But people from Asian countries, as well as Eastern European nations, must learn entirely different forms of alphabets in addition to new words with unusual sounds and grammar rules.

What does this mean for someone entering school in the United States? For many, being thrust into a class with those who know English means they must work twice as hard to become literate. They may speak one language at home and be expected to speak English at school. Moreover, they never had the same background experiences as classmates born locally. Language development, cultural norms, and communication styles growing up may be totally unfamiliar from what English learners are now facing, which puts them at a disadvantage for learning.[5]

To help someone learn English (or if you are learning a new language), try to make the words relevant to his or her (or your) interests. Boost language by transcribing a song, for example, from a CD. Or read a movie script while watching that movie. Listen to each word. Notice sentence structure, vocabulary, and slang expressions in addition to what is stressed. All these factors help someone get a feel for meaning.

Another helpful activity involves finding an e-pal to chat with online. The more anyone writes, the easier it becomes. Similarly, check out free online language courses. Or watch a video or taped television show. Listen to what is happening, and watch nonverbal communication for clues about meaning. Write down a summary of the show. Try to decipher different parts of speech or make a list

"Whether it is a pregnant pause or even talking with her hands, a debater has many expressive tricks in her repertoire, some of which may cover a multitude of sins against language. In writing, however, one's words stand naked on the page. . . . My English was weak: my sentences were often fragments; my tenses erratic; and my grammar often just not grammatical. If I could have seen it myself, I would have fixed it, but what was wrong sounded right to me. . . . I had no idea I sounded so much like my mother! . . . I bought some grammar handbooks and . . . a stack of vocabulary booklets. Over summer vacations . . . I'd devote each day's lunch hour to grammar exercises and to learning ten new words."—Supreme Court justice Sonia Sotomayor, writing about her college classwork[c]

of strange words from the show to check in the dictionary. The value of tapes is you can rewind and replay them. Learning a new language doesn't have to be all drudgery.

What's in a Name?

Students who regularly speak a language other than English and require special assistance at school are labeled various names, depending on state and federal policies. The common term for students from other countries used to be English as a second language (ESL) learners. Then the government wrote guidelines for what it now calls ELL, for English language learners. There are also dual language learners. In California, school systems prefer ELD for English language deficient. The ELD label indicates that students qualify for these programs by testing deficient, or somehow lacking, in their first language as well as English. Not a very positive approach!

Whichever the label, speech therapists strive in the same way to help their students build vocabulary and adapt to the new community. Students new to the United States go through a learning curve, just as U.S.-born citizens would living in another country. At first, they mainly listen because they cannot understand or speak. Remember this is not because they are shy or think they are better than you are: it just means they don't know enough language yet to feel comfortable talking.

As someone enters conversations, they may use gestures more. They may make mistakes or mix words from their first language with English. As they learn more words and gain confidence and fluency in their English, they may say correct words but with grammar errors. With time, conversation inches toward the level of native speakers.

How Schools Teach Students Who Speak Another Language

Too often, new immigrants receive a misdiagnosis. They might be denied certain education opportunities by being placed in special education programs that do not suit their needs.[6] Students from other countries may merely need a boost in the English language department. Luckily, many schools recognize that other programs better suit students who want to learn and improve their English.

Students who need to learn English find varying types of classes. The most frequent programs involve bilingual and ESL classes. But there are many variations of these alternatives, depending upon the goals for learners and funding within the school district.

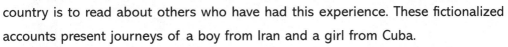

Good Reads about Teen Immigrants

A good way to better understand what it's like to suddenly be thrust into surviving in another country is to read about others who have had this experience. These fictionalized accounts present journeys of a boy from Iran and a girl from Cuba.

Borderline (HarperTeen, 2010) by Allan Stratton is a novel about Sami, a fifteen-year-old Iranian boy who comes to the United States to escape persecution in his country. Because he speaks differently and practices his family's Muslim faith, Sami experiences bullying in his new home. But his problems multiply when his father is accused of participating in a terrorist plot, and the racism escalates.

The Red Umbrella (Yearling, 2011) by Christina Diaz Gonzalez is a historical novel about fourteen-year-old Lucia Avarez, who journeyed from Cuba to America in the early 1960s. The Cuban Socialist Revolution is in full swing when Lucia and her brother become 2 of the 14,000 children sent to the United States as part of Operation Pedro Pan. Lucia winds up living in a small Nebraska farm town with an older couple. The two children try to adapt to a new language and culture at a time when they are wrestling with coming-of-age issues every teen experiences.

Bilingual Classes

One option for new immigrants who know little English is placement in a bilingual education class. The setting segregates those who have little English but speak the same language. The emphasis of bilingual education is on strengthening the original language before attempting to learn more English.

Bilingual classes are taught by someone who usually speaks the language that is learned back home. Most lessons are taught in the home language, too. Bilingual teachers usually provide some English instruction in academics. But the real goal is to strengthen skills in both the native language and English, rather than academic progress. The ultimate goal, however, is to gradually provide experiences with other students who are mainstream.

One negative with a bilingual setting is that it separates students from classmates. For some teens, this segregation slows their adapting and meeting others in school. But some students find this separation a positive. The setting allows

> "My cousin Miriam . . . was studying for a degree in bilingual education. . .
> and today is no less passionate about that calling with decades of teaching
> experience behind her. 'I want to become the kind of teacher that I wish
> I'd had,' she told me. She'd had it rough in the public schools, where the
> teachers knew so little of Latino culture they didn't realize that kids who
> looked down when scolded were doing so out of respect, as they'd been
> taught. Their gesture only invited a further scolding: 'Look at me when I
> speak to you!'"—Supreme Court justice Sonia Sotomayor[d]

them to adjust at a slower pace. They may value being integrated more gradually into a school with large numbers of students who speak a strange language, which can be overwhelming. Students often find comfort in coming to class with others who only speak their language.

If students in bilingual classes have problems adjusting to a new school and community, they feel less anxious talking with a teacher who speaks their language. But if someone cannot acquire English, or if they speak English poorly and have difficulty with academics taught in their original language, this might indicate the need for referral to someone who can test for language disabilities.

ELL Classes

Many educators—and parents—prefer students to obtain more exposure to English in an academic way. They believe more frequent exposure, when handled correctly by knowledgeable teachers and with support, provides quicker language adjustment. This happens in an ELL or ESL class.

With ELL, students learn in a regular classroom with others who speak English. But they receive assistance from a trained, certified teacher or speech therapist who works on the same material as is taught in class. This material is adapted in a way students can understand, no matter what their language.

Some ELL students gain extra support by leaving their regular class to spend part of their day with a teacher trained to work with non-English-speaking students. The class focuses on grammar, vocabulary, and communication skills. The speech teacher may be the only English speaker in the room. Academic content is usually left for the regular classroom, unless the student has specific questions. Sometimes, an aide or teacher stays in the mainstream classroom during certain academic activities. Their job is to explain projects and translate and support class seatwork and homework assignments.

> ### Teen Tip
>
> Embarrassed to be pulled from class for speech therapy? Don't be. But if you feel funny or are teased for leaving the room, request your therapy time during study hall or another situation when your leaving won't be so noticeable. It's common to become more self-conscious with age. This, too, will pass once you gain more confidence in yourself—and your speech and language skills.

Variations

School districts offer a range of options between the two main types of language classes. Some only provide what's called Early Exit Transitional classes. With these, the main goal is to teach English quickly, so students can enter mainstream classes with English-speaking teens as soon as possible. This means experiencing speedy English immersion activities rather than spending time learning academics.

How well this type of program works for a student depends upon the degree of English that person already knows. If a teen has absolutely no English skills, this type of program can be overwhelming. But if the teen speaks some English and is a quick learner, such a program might get that person comfortable at school earlier.

Some districts organize classes designed to increase knowledge in two languages. Everything is taught by two different teachers. One teacher is fluent in the foreign language, and one teaches in English.

Gabriella's Story

Gabriella doesn't have pets in America. She says her landlord doesn't allow pets in the apartment. In Mexico, Gabriella raised many different pets. She lived in a big house, she says, like a palace. She describes her place here as small.

Gabriella was worried and excited to move to Texas. She didn't know anyone there, and she didn't know how to do things other kids did. At first, she was so scared. She says her worst time was when she started high school. She couldn't finish homework because everything was in English. She had no idea what anyone was talking about.[e]

A Film about Language

Maria Jarmel and Ken Schneider produced the award-winning film *Speaking in Tongues* (www.pbs.org/programs/speaking-in-tongues, 2010) to counter negative images of people who speak differently. The film follows four families who are Chinese American, African American, Mexican American, and European American. They work to address community barriers by becoming bilingual and not just English speaking. In the process of learning someone else's language, they became bicultural as well. They learned to appreciate another culture by getting to know families and traditions from that culture. The filmmakers believe "language is a metaphor for the barriers that come between neighbors, be they across the street or around the world."[f]

When Communication Turns Biased

On July 7, 2013, an airplane from Asian Airlines, a Korean passenger carrier, crashed in San Francisco. The terrible crash killed two people and wounded several others. The next day the *Chicago Sun-Times* ran a front-page story with the title "Fright 214," a play on Flight 214 for the scheduled travel. Some headline writer must have thought it was clever to substitute the letter *r* for *l* as some Asians might pronounce the letter. But to Asian Americans, the headline proved insulting. Within twenty-four hours, the publisher apologized for the racially biased wording. But the error showed how many people work from stereotypes that come from language. Many new immigrants encounter this form of taunting daily.

Such stereotyping leads some people who can afford it to seek private speech therapy. New arrivals to the United States or those from homes where a language other than English is spoken may choose to alter their word and letter pronunciation. And stereotyping doesn't stop with newcomers. Many teens from different walks of life experience prejudice simply because of how they pronounce their words.

Debate over Different Forms of English

Many professors believe that language is the main way to transmit culture. Language develops as our society progresses in history, economy, and politics. What

Language and Politics

Educators take into account the political and cultural factors that define language versus dialect. For example, seven languages are spoken in China. Mandarin is the official national language, but Cantonese is the one spoken by a large portion of the population outside Shanghai. Speakers of either language cannot understand each other. Yet, they are from a common nation and culture. But Serbians and Croatians, although they understand one another, use their own alphabets and come from separate countries. The idea of what to call language can get dicey.

you say and how you say it expresses ideas about how you think, including about race.[7]

Prejudiced views about language extend to people born and raised in this country, many for generations. Like it or not, language and how it is spoken often determines what others think of you. If you want to be part of a certain group in school, you tend to talk like them.

During the 1980s preteen and teen girls started talking the way popular culture portrayed teens from California. A 1982 Frank Zappa song called "Valley Girl" was meant to make fun of spoiled young women who were more interested in shopping, appearance, and popularity than personal achievement. The next year, 1983, the Nicholas Cage movie *Valley Girl* brought the caricature into full view, depicting status-seeking females from the San Fernando Valley near Los Angeles. Thereafter, the name "Valley Girl" as a term for a ditz gained popularity. Valley Girls introduced words, such as "like" and "ya know," into common parlance and a way of sing-song speaking. Many viewed those who spoke that way as airheaded and unprofessional. As these teens have become radio and television reporters today, many older listeners have difficulty believing what these women say.

Speaking the same as other teens—or anyone—is a way to connect with each other and a specific culture and heritage. The same is true of people who speak regional dialects, such as individuals from the mountains of Appalachia. These traditions are important to continue. But how do these forms of English affect learning to write and read, since sounds and words are based on Standard English? How do you justify speaking a certain way that gives students a sense of pride yet may hamper their future, entry into higher education, and chances at corporate management—if they choose these manners of speaking?

Ambassador for Gullah: Candice Glover

When Candice Glover won the twelfth season of television's talent show *American Idol*, she made more than a name for herself. She shined a spotlight on her hometown of Beaufort, South Carolina, and the Gullah Geechee culture that thrives there. The Gullah people are descendants of former slaves from the rice-growing region of West Africa. Slave traders kidnapped and brought them to the United States to cultivate rice along the eastern coast of South Carolina, especially on the swampy Sea Islands, and in Georgia. Because the slaves were isolated by geography and maintained a strong culture, their heritage persisted.

Gullah language is the glue that binds the community. Until the 1940s, language specialists mistook Gullah for a form of broken English. But in 1949, Dr. Lorenzo Turned published groundbreaking research that confirmed Gullah was an official language. People who speak Gullah blend several African languages, mainly from present-day Sierra Leone, with Creole and English. They use distinct rhythms, accents, and words to sing and speak, all the while keeping their heritage alive. With a common vocabulary and grammar, Gullah transmits cultural traditions, songs, history.

Candace Glover may be one of the younger Gullah to achieve stardom. But she is not alone. Supreme Court justice Clarence Thomas, who grew up in Pin Point, Georgia, spoke Gullah. So did South Carolina's congressman James Clyburn. As author Dr. Emory Campbell wrote in his *Gullah Cultural Legacies*, "The Gullah language more than any other cultural asset has allowed Gullah people to remain in one big family."[9]

When Talking Reflects Culture

Every culture teaches children to hold certain values. These values often guide how someone communicates within and outside the community. Native Americans, for example, place great emphasis on community and the tribal structure.[8] As such, they value cooperation and harmony within groups above individual efforts.

Because the group is so important within the community, elders stress modesty, even when someone achieves high goals. Many native children are taught to remain quiet and to wait patiently. Not the usual fare in today's immediate, frenetic society. Similarly, some never waste words, meaning they rarely chatter for

The Talking Stick

One Native American tradition that crosses cultural—and communication—borders is called the talking stick. Although part of some Native American cultures for centuries, teachers use the method to improve cross-cultural understanding in ELL classrooms.[h]

Native Americans have employed the talking stick as a way to ensure that an individual can speak without interruption during tribal and council meetings. The elder speaks first without interruption. Then the elder passes the stick to the next person in the circle and so on around until everyone who chooses gets a turn to speak. Others are required to listen intently until the stick comes to them. What every speaker says has equal value.

The talking stick works in class much the same way. The Teacher sits students in a circle and hands the stick to one person to begin. The student holding the stick speaks uninterrupted until finished and then hands the stick to the next person. No judgments. No comments on what is said. No talking all at once—or until the speaker selects the next person to talk. Listeners are to do just that—listen to the student holding the stick without figuring out what they will say when it is their turn.

Teachers who use the talking stick believe students feel heard and understood. The experience gives them active participation in learning instead of the teacher always lecturing. If the teacher presents certain issues, everyone has their say, no matter how controversial. A version of the talking stick would work for family or group meetings, too. What better way to build communication bridges than to feel you are respected?

the sake of talking. When someone expresses an idea or feeling, they often speak slowly and deliberately to convey the power of what they are saying.

Because many Native American students tend to speak in a thoughtful manner, they may seem shy or disinterested. Non-Native Americans may find them unfriendly. Teachers may interpret the lack of responses to questions or verbal participation in group projects or discussions as a sign of limited intelligence.

Therefore, understanding where someone comes from in terms of background and culture is important to communicating—and learning—in a meaningful way.

Modifying Accents

This heading is misleading. Why? Because according to the American Speech-Language-Hearing Association (ASHA), "everyone speaks with an accent." ASHA defines an accent as the distinctive way each person speaks the same language.

Accent comes as result of the U.S. region where teens live or their country of origin. Sometimes teens assume characteristics of their parents' accents without even knowing. For example, someone born in the United States whose father originally came from Poland may leave off word endings or say the initial word sound *d* for *th*. The person sounds more like his old-world father than someone from the family's current neighborhood.

Accents are most obvious when moving to another region of the country. People who grew up in Chicago and moved to Louisville, Kentucky, may suddenly start adding "y'all" to conversations. Their heavier Chicago *a* sound may turn into a softer southern *ah*. People rarely realize they are picking up these regional ways of talking, but it happens all the time in a salad bowl culture.

While accents are not a speech or language disorder, they can cause problems with communication. For example, if you studied Spanish in high school, you may not be able to understand someone who speaks Spanish and is from Spain. A Spaniard speaks a variation of Spanish that someone from Mexico or Guatemala may not understand.

If your strong accent doesn't jibe with your current community, you may find others do not understand you. Or you may limit conversations because you feel unheard and misunderstood and hate repeating yourself. You may worry about undue attention the accent causes. This is especially problematic if speaking affects job performance, participating in class, or meeting people socially.

Changing a Foreign Accent

Changing an accent requires hard work, but it's not impossible. One therapist estimates that articulation exercises need to be practiced two minutes a day at least three times a week to change sound production. Many clients may find being consistent difficult. But if teens are willing to put in the time and practice to make changes, a speech therapist can help alter how they sound.

During a speech evaluation, students will be asked to read passages aloud. From the reading, the therapist analyzes how they pronounce sounds and the

---

Mike's Story

Mike was raised in New York City where "all kinds of people are mixed together." He went to school where they all spoke Standard English, although many with a New York accent. Mike didn't have one, though, because his parents spoke without a trace of Black English, as far as he knew. Just before Mike turned thirteen, his family moved to Charlotte, North Carolina. He went to a private school until he begged to go to public school. The school was all black. And there he was with a New York accent. And he was entering puberty. Mike remembers longing to fit in. So, he started talking like the other boys. He dropped the letter *g* off the ends of words and started constructing sentences with double negatives like his classmates. Mike says his parents went ballistic when he spoke like that at home. He ended that way of talking quickly, although he still got teased at school.[i]

---

rhythm and tone of how they speak. Once specific sounds and patterns are documented, the therapist can suggest exercises to reduce or modify the offending sounds.

Graduate students from other nations who teach at Ohio University spend about two hours a day, sometimes for up to a year, perfecting their American English.[9] They are motivated to change how they speak because their accents are preventing professional growth. With one in six graduate students from another country, universities are finally addressing what undergraduates have been complaining about for years: the inability to understand their teachers, many of whom are graduate students from other lands. Other professors complain they cannot understand their colleagues. In addition to special classes, some universities require applicants from outside the United States to take the Test of English as a Foreign Language.[10] This test and other software programs have listening and speaking components that analyze speech.

Altering Regional Accents

Therapists see clients for a variety of reasons relating to accent. Some people from other countries want to minimize obvious speech that targets them as newcomers. They want to sound more American. Others want to limit sounds from their former community, such as rid themselves of a Midwest twang or southern drawl. On a few occasions, students choose to alter their speech, for example, if they are

> "I have several adult clients who want to alter their regional accents. One client lived in the Midwest for fifteen years before she was finally ready to make some changes. She said she was tired of sounding like singer and actress Bette Midler and not earning her money. The client was originally from the Bronx section of New York City. When you move to a certain culture, it's hard to avoid sounding the way the locals do."
> —Suzi Shulman, long-time speech therapist.[j]

teased for a hissing *s* or whiny sounds. Professionals often choose to reduce their regional accents to sound more worldly. And actors want more universal sounding speech, so they have a chance to be chosen for more diverse roles.

Nonverbal Communication and Social Pragmatics

Another important communication issue involves the missteps that can result from gestures, touching, and other verbal and nonverbal communications that vary among cultures. Eye contact that means teens are paying attention to a speaker in the United States may be considered rude or disrespectful in many Asian countries. Similarly, Russians on the street or a bus rarely smile at each other because others might think them unusual. Hugging and kissing among men that is common in Arab countries may seem out of place to certain uptight, macho men from the United States.

Even the distance between speaking partners means something special culturally. Standing very close when talking can be a sign of intimacy, which is not always welcome. But being too far away, especially in Latin American countries, can be perceived as unfriendly. Taking turns or talking over someone else can indicate where someone originates. Animated discussions with everyone talking at once or arms flailing is more accepted in some communities than others.

These types of communications are part of what speech therapists call *social pragmatics*. Social pragmatics are the unspoken standards that govern behaviors for social interactions. Even if you know a language and speak clearly, you may still miss the subtle variations in how thoughts should be communicated. You may fail to grasp the complexity of social communications in certain situations. Or you may lack the sensitivity to know when and in what way or situation to say it.

Adapting Socially Has No Age Limit

Even highly educated older newcomers have problems adjusting to a new land. "It took years to get adjusted," microbiologist Jan Vilcek told the *New York Times* about his coming to the United States from Germany in the 1980s. "Although I spoke English, understanding accents was difficult. We could communicate, but we often didn't know what people were talking about. And there were matters of social interaction that were puzzling—a cocktail party. We'd never been to a cocktail party."[k]

Exploring Social Pragmatics

Social pragmatics are the cultural communication rules—behaviors, attitudes, and policies—that you usually pick up automatically as you mature. For example, you know not to tell a joke during a funeral service. Or you never shout at another person in a quiet theater. These situations are somewhat obvious. But someone from another culture may not understand the subtle language involved in less obvious social interactions. Slang or joking phrases that are part of one society may be taken at their word and totally misunderstood in another culture. To someone first learning English, these sensitivities need to be specifically taught. They go along with building vocabulary during individual or group therapy sessions.

According to the ASHA, pragmatics covers three main social communication skills.[11] One is how you know to use language for different purposes. For example, you speak to request something ("I need new shoes.") or greet someone ("Hey!" or "See you later!"). Or you share information through language, such as "The burner is still hot." These situations involve the ability to request information in return, such as clarifying unclear messages or asking someone to expand on the topic being discussed.

Another skill that is important with social communication is how you alter your language depending upon the listener and situation. For example, some people talk to babies in a higher pitch than their regular voice. If you talked like that to other teenagers, they would think you are either making fun of them or treating them like a baby. In another example, you probably speak differently in the locker room with classmates than you would at a formal family gathering or religious service. Or you should!

The most sensitive pragmatic skill to learn covers rules for general conversation and storytelling. This can be tricky because it involves following the set of rules that varies most among cultures. Taking turns while conversing, standing near or far enough from the other person, using hand gestures and eye contact or not—these depend upon the situation and culture. And they can get you into trouble with your conversation partner, if you get it wrong.

Social Pragmatics and Other Language Problems

Social pragmatics also come into play with individuals who have autism or other communication impairment. These conditions often leave individuals without certain knowledge of social awareness. Brain injury is another situation that may interfere with the normal filters that allow people to adapt during everyday social situations. Any complex concept—such as verbal slang, metaphors (words that represent something else), and idioms (local sayings)—can be confusing. Body language or different perspectives, moods, or values can cause inappropriate responses.

For example, teens without the filter to moderate their voice or what they say may blurt out, possibly yelling, anything on their minds at the time, no matter how hurtful. For example, you usually do not tell someone that their clothes are ugly. In another example, teens with autism may be so focused on what they want

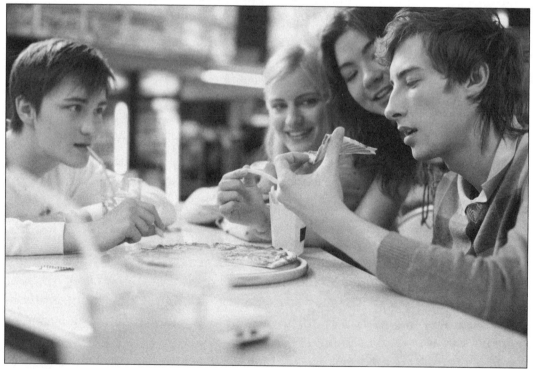

Teen checks out a different type of food, pizza, with the help of friends.

at the time they may not understand that action *now* is impossible. Any attempt to delay might provoke a tantrum and screaming.

Difficulties with social pragmatics may appear as inappropriate topics during conversation or talk that veers way off topic. For example, individuals with attention problems often have trouble focusing during a conversation. They may easily be distracted by anything around them. They may suddenly notice and read a sign in the middle of a conversation about current events. Someone might tell long, rambling stories that make no sense to listeners or say the same thing repeatedly without seeming to notice—or care.

Speech therapists may notice a problem with social language during a specific time, such as when teens are nervous. But if a therapist observes that a student consistently communicates in an inappropriate manner for his or her age, the therapist or teacher can request testing for a pragmatic disorder. The disorder can be in addition to another language problem, such as autism or learning disabilities, or be independent. Speech and language therapy in individual and group sessions can help replace social awkwardness with awareness of helpful social skills.

Helping Someone with A Social Pragmatic Challenge

The best way to assist teens who have a social pragmatic challenge is to include them in as many activities as possible. That way, they learn language, cultural rules, and how to behave. Teens without pragmatic challenges need to understand what is involved in these seemingly ordinary outings.

Take eating out, for instance. In some countries, such as Peru or Togo, or in some U.S. families, young people never experience restaurants. Socially challenged teens may find the give-and-take of communicating with a waitress puzzling. What do terms, such as *entree* or *dessert*, on the menu mean? Tipping rules vary with the country. In some places, such as in many European nations, a percentage of the total is added to the bill for service. But in the United States, the wait staff expects extra money as a tip. Different amounts indicate pleasure or displeasure with service. There are so many situations U.S. teens take for granted that someone from another background has to specifically learn. And everyone learns better through experience.

Therefore, you can help someone with a language disorder learn social skills by going places together. During these instances, you constantly verbalize what is correct and incorrect about the situation or activity. You can ask your friend with limited speech questions. After hearing responses, try to respond with complete thoughts, so the other person hears you model correct grammar and pronunciation and in appropriate ways.

Invisible Written Languages

Research shows that students from other countries learn new concepts best in their native language. But what if their first language has no written form? How can teachers find materials? How can students improve their native language skills?

More than 6,000 of the 6,800 languages are spoken by less than a million people. A small percentage of languages belong to communities of less than 1,000 speakers.[l] Such small communities are more likely than larger regions to speak a language without a written form, such as the Zoroastrian Mobeds in India.[m]

Without a formal writing system, people from these communities often remain sidelined. They cannot communicate in a lasting way with each other and with people in other communities. The effects can be political, limiting power to exchange ideas. Lack of ability to communicate can influence the local economy when merchants have no way to exchange goods outside their village, limiting income. For students entering the United States, the effects can be educational. Without knowledge of written language, students are restricted in what they can learn. They cannot exchange ideas with others far away or in a lasting form. How can their community retain and share information for future generations?

If outings are impossible, create role-playing situations at home. For example, pretend to be different people, such as a salesperson in a store or an elderly person, to encourage varying language. You can ask your friend to tell a story about something, either made up or something from life in their country of origin. Encourage gestures, changes in facial expression, anything that will embellish the story and provide more information to you.

Written Language

Written language allows us to see words in a material form. In fact, teachers tell new readers that writing is really talk written down. Through writing, readers learn how to combine words to organize and make sense of verbal language. Sounds and words develop into written sentences and paragraphs.

Written language tends to be more complex than spoken language. It follows certain rules of grammar, punctuation, and placement of clauses. With speaking, you can say incomplete sentences, repeat something, or take it back. You have the benefit of gestures, like pointing, or facial expressions to complete thoughts.

Written language helps you communicate, socialize, and share cultural values and information. You write letters (so retro), books, magazines, newspapers, and now electronic media with computers, smart phones, social networks, e-mails, texts, and blogs. These forms tend to be more permanent than a fleeting conversation, at least until the computer program crashes. There is more time to mull over what you write and eliminate slang words, such as *like* or *you know*. Still, written language can be a huge problem for anyone unfamiliar with English.

For teens challenged by English and writing, a good place to begin improving is to plan what to say first. Deciding on format helps ensure that readers will be able to follow the logic of what you are trying to convey. Here is where pragmatics may be helpful. For example, someone new to English may want to construct a report. Does the teacher prefer certain formats? What phrases are acceptable and absolutely unacceptable? Look for similar writing examples to imitate. Once you determine how to organize the project, begin writing with words you already know. You know them because you can say them in conversation. Check for missing words in the dictionary or with computer spell check.

Never assume your writing is correct the first time around. Teachers always tell students to revise. Whether you are writing in a dominant or a different language, revision is a given. Many times the author cannot see errors, so ask someone else to check grammar. Arrange with the teacher to offer feedback as the writing project progresses.

Misspelling will happen. So will grammatical errors, especially when English isn't your main language. One way to help decrease the number of misspellings is to keep a log. When you see one or several words that cause continual grief, you may notice a pattern. For example, someone from Japan may spell words with *r* instead of *l* because there is no *l* in the Japanese alphabet. Or you may use pronouns irregularly. A log would indicate something to focus on to correct future spelling or grammar problems.

Beyond the log, specifically study grammar rules and compare how they are different from or similar to a first language. As an example, English speakers capitalize formal names but not all nouns. For another example, Americans capitalize names such as *Mary* or *Michael*, but not names for objects such as *desk* or *glasses*. Germans, however, write an initial capital for all nouns, such as *Sohn* (son) or *Stadt* (city).

Some grammar rules fall under the heading of social pragmatism even with writing. Therefore, you need to follow certain cultural rules to learn what is

Reading Written Language

Part of learning another language—and perfecting the one normally used—is knowing how to read for information and pleasure. Reading fluently is one of the most difficult, and at times embarrassing, aspects of second language learning. What if you are asked to read aloud? What if you cannot understand directions to locate the paragraph, complete a task at work, or answer questions on a quiz?

According to Shari Roberson, professor of speech-language pathology at Indiana University of Pennsylvania, reading fluency involves "the ability to read text accurately, smoothly, and rapidly. These factors build the ability to comprehend meaning from written words."[n] Roberson suggests certain strategies to improve reading competence:

- Select reading materials that fit your reading level, rather than your age. Librarians and teachers can help select books that are especially prepared for older readers but do not look like baby books with lots of pictures. Usually, these books are about topics teens might like, just written for those unfamiliar with a range of words.
- Look at punctuation, which helps you know when to pause or when the thought is complete. Underline words that might benefit from emphasizing, such as "*Help!*" or "I *want* that." Would the meaning be different if emphasis was on "*I* want that" or "I want *that*"? Read with a trusted friend or teacher to receive assistance.
- Choose stories that are similar to others you have already read. That way, you can build on the words and some information you already know.
- Locate old movie scripts online to read, particularly ones for movies you have seen. Recall how actors said the words and in what context, which increases your ability to read fluently.

considered acceptable or rude in different cultures. In Russia, punctuation rules are far more important than in the United States. Learning the particulars of any language can be difficult. Add grammar rules and appropriateness to specific situations, and it's a wonder anyone becomes bilingual and multilingual—in speaking or writing.

Resources

Organizations

Gullah Heritage Consulting Services
P.O. Box 22136
Hilton Head, SC 29926
843-681-7066
www.gullaheritage.com
Home for information about the Gullah people, culture, and language, and publisher of the foremost book about Gullah, *Gullah Cultural Legacies*.

National Association for Bilingual Education
8701 Georgia Avenue, Suite 700
Silver Spring, MD 20910
240-450-3700
www.nabe.org
A national organization devoted to being a resource and advocate for bilingual learners and bilingual education professionals, including publishing a journal and hosting conferences.

National Clearinghouse for English Language Acquisition
2011 Eye Street NW, Suite 300
Washington, DC 20006
800-321-6223
www.ncela.gwu.edu
Organization authorized by the federal government as a resource to help teachers and students who are dealing with or are English language learners.

Patchworks Films
663 7th Avenue
San Francisco, CA 94118
800-343-5540
www.patchworkfilms.com

Film and production company responsible for the award-winning documentary *Speaking in Tongues* that is shown in schools, museums, and libraries as a positive educational tool to build acceptance of everyone who speaks another language.

Penn Center
P.O. Box 126
16 Penn Center Circle West
St. Helena Island, SC 29920
843-838-2474
www.penncenter.com
Historical and cultural landmark district of nineteen buildings that house a museum, historical documents, and conference center renowned for Gullah and southern black cultures.

WIDA (World-Class Instructional Design and Assessment)
Housed in Wisconsin Center for Education Research
School of Education, University of Wisconsin
Madison, WI 53706
866-276-7735
www.wida.us
Up-to-date research and resources and activities to advance language development and standards and academic achievement for preschool through grade 12 for English language learners.

TECHNOLOGY AS A COMMUNICATION GAME CHANGER

The ability to communicate remains one of your most important tools to interact with the world. In your parents' generation that meant talking face-to-face, telephoning by turning rotary dials on landlines, and writing letters to mail, as in snail mail. Then technology comes along and transforms how everyone relates to one another.

Instant messages and photos. No face-to-face contact. Not needing to talk with someone verbally. Don't want to communicate with a contact? Simple, just click them gone. What could be easier? This is especially true for teens who have trouble communicating for any reason—a speech and language disorder, different means of communicating, or choice to keep self-expression to a minimum. Admit it: the ever-changing parade of new technology devices has been a boon for teen communication.

Technology in general plays an expanding and significant role in every aspect of life. In the United States, individuals conduct business, government, and education online. That's in addition to fostering overall communication just to chat, socialize, and locate information. Young people rarely use maps, calculators, or dictionaries anymore. Why? You don't have to with GPS systems, smartphones, and spell checking. In its 2013 report, the National Dissemination Center for Children with Disabilities calculates that technology has had an impact on the lives of more than 50 million people with disabilities alone.[1]

Connected Teens

So what technology suits your communication needs? The answer for most teens seems to be everything. The Pew Research Center, an online fact center that produces unbiased polls and research, verifies what every teen already knows.

"I have had my own laptop since eighth grade. That way, I can write papers without bothering my parents. I have an iPhone and an iPad for school, which I don't use that much. And I watch television. For social media I'm on Facebook, Twitter, Instagram, Tumblr, Pinterest, YouTube, and Snapchat. I used Facebook a lot in junior high and sent pictures through Instagram. Now I send videos with Pinterest and YouTube and take pictures and send them to people through Snapchat. With the cell phone, I mostly text or play games. My phone is with me 95 percent of the time. I go on Pinterest, text, or look up people. I love watching on Netflix."
— Kaylee, high school junior, on technology[a]

Technology usage is not only frequent but on the rise, especially with teens and young adults.[2]

According to a September 2012 Pew survey, 95 percent of all teens between twelve and seventeen years are online. That's the same rate as the next age range, the eighteen- to twenty-nine-year-old crowd. In addition, 78 percent of teens own cell phones, with 47 percent of them being smartphones. And these phones are increasingly being used to send and receive text messages. Between 2008 and 2009 alone, the number of teens who sent text messages almost doubled from 38 percent to 54 percent.[3]

A huge number of Internet users (93 percent) have access to computers. Eight in ten teens own a desktop or laptop. Most often these are shared among family members. Of the other 20 percent of teens without their own computer, two-thirds find one at home to use.[4]

Numbers are also large for joining social media sites. Eighty-one percent of connected teens access some type of social media. Although new social media appear regularly, Facebook still commands 77 percent of online teen activity.[5] A typical teen claims about 300 friends.

Most teens create basic profiles on social networks. They include name, age, photo of themselves, and interests. Fewer post school names (73 percent), towns where they live (72 percent), relationship status (3 percent), e-mail address (54 percent), and videos of themselves (25 percent).[6] The scariest figure is the increase from 2 percent to 20 percent in the number of teens who share cell phone numbers on social media.[7]

Usually, teens post messages as a way to communicate with people on their approved friend list. They arrange social activities and sometimes flirt. But one

When Is Too Much Too Much?

Mathias Crawford, researcher at Stanford University, wants to know how much technology is too much. He studies human-computer interactions and communications. Crawford found that "every experience is being mediated and conceived around how it can be captured and augmented by our devices. No place is this more apparent than our meals. . . . People make dinner reservations on Opentable, check in on Foursquare when they arrive at the restaurant, take a picture of their food to share on Instagram, post on Twitter a joke they hear during the meal, review the restaurant on Yelp, then coordinate a ride home using Uber."[b]

Pew survey found that about 50 percent of teens use social media to engage new friends.[8]

Twitter, for those living in a cave, is that online social networking service that allows users to send and read text-based messages, or tweets, that contain up to only 140 characters. First started in 2006 in San Francisco, by 2012 Twitter handled more than 500 million registered users worldwide. Users send an average of 340 million tweets per day. One hundred forty million users are from the United States. By the end of 2012, 26 percent of teens had opened Twitter accounts, and the number keeps growing.[9] Other social media sites do not compare to Facebook or Twitter in numbers, potential numbers, or growth patterns—at least not yet.

Fair and Balanced Assessments

Even with so many benefits, there are pros and cons to relying on devices to communicate. Illinois speech therapist Suzi Shulman sees both sides in her private practice and working with students in schools:

> I think e-mail helps people's writing skills, but texting ruins them. With e-mail, people exchange ideas more, and they learn to spell check. They write on a regular basis, where they might not write otherwise. As with anything, practice improves the idea of creating something with words and writing it down. But with texting, everything is shorter. Texters use abbreviated spelling and cut corners with grammar.
>
> Both affect social skills. Some people use language less often because they're writing instead of speaking. Or they are so busy texting that they

The Joys of E-mailing

Sure, e-mail is easy and convenient. Writing and sending an e-mail often takes much less time than calling a chatty friend or family member. And sending a message via e-mail means you don't have to hear the reader's exclamation or anger at the other end. For anyone who sends a response you don't like, just click Delete. Couldn't get much easier.

Problems arise when way too many e-mails zip up and back in different time frames over the same minor issue. Difficulties multiply when several people are involved, which really throws off timing. Or you send a message, then think of something else that's important to include. The addition requires yet another e-mail that someone probably won't read until after they responded to your first one. Very confusing.

With e-mail—or texting and social media—you cannot get an accurate reaction to what you have written. At times, so many communications go up and back, some friends throw up their hands and write: *This isn't working. Call me!*

don't talk with each other. People who rely on other, technical forms of communication can't help but experience changes. Language is like anything else: if you don't use it, you lose it.[10]

California speech therapist Christy Cook agrees that the benefits of technology are a mixed bag:

Technology has definitely changed communication styles. For some on the autism spectrum, it opens the door to relating. Teens with autism may not look at a person, but they will look at a digital representation. They will interact with a computer program but not with a teacher.

Overall I've noticed that students don't know how to write. They talk in techspeak and prefer instant gratification. My colleagues and I often argue about whether a child has ADHD or is a victim of technology. Does the student have behaviors that result from bombardment of everything or a serious medical ADHD diagnosis?

E-mailing on computers came into use when I was in college. For the most part, I and my friends typed papers on typewriters, revised, and typed all over again. A lot of young people today are not good spellers because they rely on spell check. Many schools have stopped teaching spelling or cursive writing because their students write on computers. Different world.[11]

Pros of Technology for Teens with a Disability

For anyone unable to speak or benefit from sign language, technology offers an array of communication alternatives. The type of device depends upon level of functioning and how this technology fits into a current communication and education program.

Before so many computer options were invented, one key communication enhancer for nontalkers was a hard copy or electronic communication board with pictures. For example, a board or chart with many small pictures, letters, and/or words would be presented. Students would point to a picture or spell words they wanted to communicate. Many times pictures looked different from the same objects at home, which limited understanding. And spelling words letter-by-letter was time-consuming.

Now computer apps offer users varied levels of programs to communicate through pictures. One option involves locating several pictures for each object quickly. Selected apps permit calling up words and learning new communication skills through a range of activities and books available online. To respond to educational software for computer programs, users simply press a color-coded Yes and No button to access higher-level concepts.

Certain children, such as Carly (see Carly's Story on page 160) and others with autism, naturally take to computers as a means of communication. Many teens like Carly often spell words on the keyboard beyond their previously perceived capabilities with writing, thinking, or communicating. Computers afford a whole new world of recreation and learning opportunities. Technology devices are unemotional and nonjudgmental. Operators are in total control because they work independently—a positive for those preteens and teens eager to do their own thing separate from adults—and at their own rate.

Computers are great equalizers. Playing computer games with others, whether they have a communication disorder or not, takes away reliance on voice. So technology becomes a bridge for socializing. Social networking sites and blogs and tweets do not require speaking, so no one has to know how well someone speaks or hears.

For teens with limited academic abilities, computer skills can translate into future jobs. Technology motivates those who might be uninterested in academic

Carly's Story

Some stories of successes with technology sound mind-boggling. Take Carly's journey with autism. She was first diagnosed at age two. Doctors told her parents not to expect learning beyond that of a six year old. Carly never talked, only made strange noises to communicate. She screamed and threw tantrums. She hit herself. She seemed in a world of her own, frustrated that she could not communicate. Her upset and upsetting behavior and lack of ability to communicate took her beyond the reach of her family. But her parents never gave up. They kept trying to reach her. They knew there was a little girl inside who longed to be heard.

When Carly was eleven years old, she had regular sessions at the computer with her speech therapist. Recently, her speech therapist had introduced activities with pictures and symbols on the computer. One day, Carly reached across the keyboard and typed "mean." Turns out she was telling her therapist that she didn't like being pushed so hard to work. Her surprised therapist asked what else Carly had to say. Then Carly typed, "Teeth hurt." These two communications put everyone on notice: there is a bright girl inside Carly's body. As Carly typed more messages, everyone discovered that this girl had feelings, emotions, the power to think critically, and lots of opinions about everything, some humorous.

Once, Carly was totally unable to communicate. Now words and thoughts spill out of her through the computer. She blossomed as the computer became her voice. "I am not able to talk out of my mouth," Carly writes on her website Carly's Voice. "However, I have found another way to communicate by spelling on my computer."[c]

In the years since that first communication, Carly and her father have written a book. It is a firsthand exchange between a witty teen and her father about what Carly's life has been like with autism. Carly has been on television, and she participates in gifted and special classes in a typical high school. She has thousands of friends on Twitter and Facebook.

But she says that one of her best achievements is the website she hosts. One page allows parents and anyone interested in autism to ask questions and have them answered by someone who knows, someone with autism. "I have a dream now," Carly, who still cannot speak with words, writes. "And that is to help people with autism find a voice."[d]

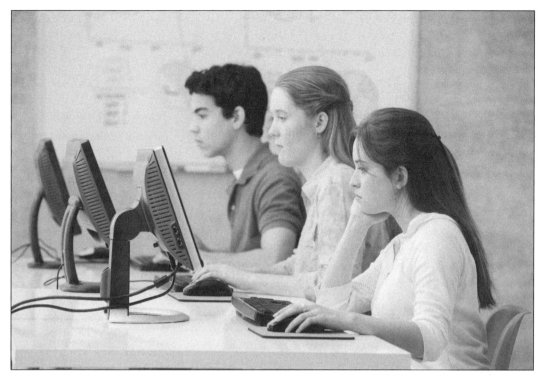

Computers—and technology in general—have been motivational as a learning tool. Research, preparing papers, taking tests, checking spelling: students can do it all online.

careers to consider computer-related adult vocational training. Teens with moderate autism can find work using computing and keyboarding skills. These jobs usually do not require social competence with face-to-face interpersonal skills.

Computers are playing a greater role in helping English language learners increase vocabulary. IPads hold hundreds of speech apps. Language programs give pictures and words and voice to enhance learning. Listening to music and talking with English-speaking friends on cell phones provides speech and language to model.

Computers host an array of apps to help with communication. Voice recognition programs allow those who cannot communicate with their voice to input messages and receive spoken feedback. New technologies for computers appear seemingly daily.

More Pros of Technology: Alternative Communication and Dysarthria

When motor problems affect someone's ability to talk, finding another means of communicating can be life changing. People who have dysarthria, a motor speech disorder, may find their articulation problems so severe that they are difficult to understand. Dysarthria involves damage to motor areas of the brain. In turn, the damage contributes to developing problems with breathing, airflow, and movement of the larynx. This damage results in poor speech quality and challenges with being understood.

When someone has difficulty expressing sounds, they are unable to socialize. As a result, their true personality winds up distorted. You can only imagine how difficult it would be to tell a joke or offer a quick quip if parts of your communication system refused to work. Alternative technology can enhance speech. Some computers have capability to speak for you. Just key in what you want to say, and the computer says it.

Availability of Communication Technology: It's the Law

Lawmakers believed technology was so important for communicating, especially for individuals with disabilities, that they enacted the Technology-Related Assistance for Individuals with Disabilities Act of 1988 (known as the Tech Act or public law 100-407). Every few years the Tech Act gets a reboot, which is a good

Technology Helps Movie Critic Regain His Mojo

In 2002, the famous journalist, film critic, and television personality Roger Ebert received a diagnosis of thyroid cancer. At first, radiation therapy helped. But four years later the cancer returned. Surgeons removed part of Ebert's lower jaw, which was traumatic. Essentially, the surgery ended his television career, eating foods he liked, and talking with friends and family. Or so the public thought.

A resourceful, determined man, Ebert returned to television. How? With the help of a computer-generated voice he controlled by his keyboard. But his voice sounded stilted, like most computer voices. A few years later, he discovered CereProc, a Scottish company that analyzes voice recordings. The company took Ebert's original voice and created computer-generated sounds closer to his original speech patterns. Voice-generated technology and computers in general allowed Ebert to continue writing for the *Chicago Sun-Times*, blogs, Facebook, and Twitter, and participate in the film review television show he created. Cancer and surgery could not stop Ebert from communicating, as long as he had the means to find a technology match. He led a full life until his death in 2013.

thing considering how quickly technology changes. Congress voted on the latest update in 2004.

Under this legislation, assistive technology covers "any item, piece of equipment, or product system . . . that is used to increase, maintain, or improve functional capabilities of individuals with disabilities."[12] The law grants funds for each U.S. state and territory to provide lifelong services to people with disabilities in their locale. Many states host centers where qualified individuals can select, adapt, repair, or replace assistive technology that helps them communicate. Teens with a communication disorder can find, try out, and borrow a range of technical equipment, including speech generating devices, voice amplifiers, speech recognition equipment, and adapted computer keyboards. Trained staff is available to help. To locate the closest local assistive technology center, go to www.resnaprojects .org/allcontacts/statewidecontacts.html.

Cons of Technology: Time Suckers

The title of a book by Alex Pang, *The Distraction Addiction*, brings up a major problem with technology. Gadgets can be so enticing that teens like you cannot stop using them. You check information. You look to see if friends have called. You investigate whatever you care about as your latest interest. Many people are simply addicted to technology—all day every day. As Pang wrote, "People who spend all day with computers used to be called hackers. Today, that's all of us."[13]

According to a 2005 Pew Research Center report, average Americans ages twelve to seventeen spend about 72.8 hours a week talking with friends via technology, such as cell phones, e-mail, instant messaging, or text messaging. That's 405.6 hours a year. In the work or school world, that would equal 50.7 eight-hour

"I'm sure I could track how much time I spend on technology, but I'd feel terrible if I did. One night I was on Pinterest two and a half hours. Some nights not at all. I know a lot of friends who are constantly checking social media in high school. I don't any more. It's distracting. Sometimes, I would come home from school and think I'll look at a site for a little while but get lost in it for a long time. Before long, time would get away from me. I had to stay up late doing homework, which made me tired the next day. Learning to balance yourself with social media is a good skill to have."

—Daniel, on technology and wasting time[e]

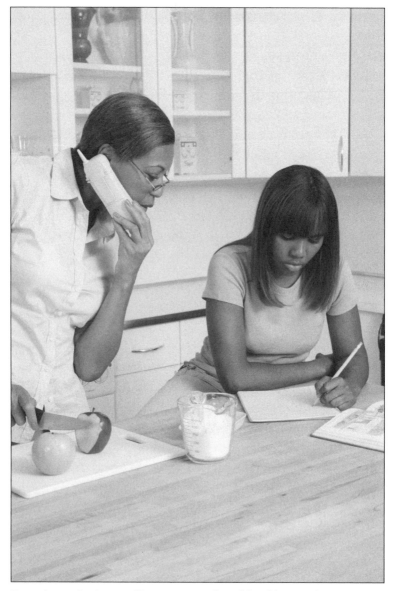

Parents are just as guilty as teens of multitasking and not paying attention. This busy mom talks on the phone, cooks, and helps her daughter with homework, or at least tries. Something has to give.

days a year, enough time for several vacations. Amount of time lost to communications through technology has increased since. And now there is texting. Fifty percent of teens send 50 or more text messages a day. An incredible one in three teens tap out more than 100 text messages a day. That's a time-sucking 3,000 messages a month! Just think of what you could accomplish in the time you take to e-mail, text, and phone friends. You could actually find friends and talk face-to-face.[14]

Toll on Family Communications

How many times have you seen a parent riding a bicycle with a youngster on the back while clicking a text message? Or another adult who pushes a buggy with a child inside while walking the dog and carrying on an animated cell phone conversation? Or the parent who allows their tweets, texts, and cell phone ringing to interrupt family discussions? Teens need their parents to be role models. When you or your parents choose technology over someone in front of you, you are saying that whoever is online matters more than the person in front of you. Time to call a family meeting, one without technology, so everyone can focus on each other.

Teens, especially girls between fourteen and seventeen, prefer to communicate with friends via text messaging. But most teens acknowledge that old-fashioned phoning works better when talking with parents and communicating sensitive

"Having technology makes it easier to communicate with family. When my parents want to know where we are, they can ask and not send police after us. My family is big on texting. If my mom needs something, she'll text. If any of us are in a quiet area, we text. But we Skype, like when I was traveling or when we want to talk with my siblings in college. That way, my parents could see we were okay and where we are supposed to be.

"When we all eat together, no one is on the phone or laptop. Sometimes, one of us would get a text, and we'd automatically go to respond. But my parents would stop us. When we're with family at any event, that's our time to communicate and catch up with them, so we turn off our phones.

"I've had experiences with kids and adults who are glued to the phone. My mom has Facebook and is technologically centered. My dad is more into television and not social media. My dad only uses the phone for texting, e-mail, and playing card games.

"Some parents limit technology for their kids. But we were never so addicted that my parents had to put limits on anything. We all have our own computers. Unless we got into trouble, which we didn't, we never had limits on technology."— Kaylee, on family communication[f]

messages to anyone. The reason is texting lacks emotion. You cannot use inflection or expression. Therefore, communications can be misunderstood in a variety of unexpected ways. You may text something you intend as a joke that is taken literally. Or you write something straight that is taken sarcastically. Best to handle sensitive topics by phone or in person.

Being plugged into technology has changed communication among many family members. Families might have less conversation around the dinner table because fingers are moving, or individuals are glued to their screens. These families might experience fewer occasions when people actually share recreation activities—that are active—because they sit in front of computer screens or bury ears in cell phones. Many people feel less creative or find less creativity all around because of reliance on computer-generated information. In some families parents feel left out of their teens' lives when they don't know and have never met friends who live online.

Addicted to Technology?

How do you know when you are hooked on technology? Take a hard look at your day. Do you switch off your alarm clock and automatically reach for the smartphone? Do you check e-mail before getting out of bed? Social media sites? Texts? Are you constantly watching for something new on the computer screen and switching from one website to another? Are you receiving and sending hundreds of messages each day, many meaningless newsletters, coupons, deals, or social media updates? Do you put off chores and homework to watch a new viral video or online movie? Do you miss appointments because you become engrossed online? Do you stay home to socialize electronically, rather than visit with friends live or go places together? When you are with friends, do you constantly interrupt what they are saying to look up the topic being discussed, rather than focus on the speaker and conversation?

If the answer is yes to any or many of these questions, chances are you better limit time spent on technology. Best to wean yourself off technology gradually. Turn off cell phones for a growing number of minutes each day. And definitely disconnect devices during meals, with friends and family, and in class.

When Is a Friend a Friend?

Many articles tackle the thorny question of whether social media has changed friendships. But first you need to seriously think about what friendship means to you. Once you define the idea of a friend and what makes a good friend, you can better evaluate how this definition compares with what goes on online.

Some journalists believe the idea of being friended is a joke, not to mention a grammatical distortion of a familiar word. They write that social media reduces communication to a popularity contest. Teens grapple with enough of that behavior at this age as it is. Why expose yourself to more on some device?

These same people worry that friending magnifies insecurities. Those of you with fewer friends might feel slighted or unpopular. Of course, this assumes that these numbers count more than the quality of friendships.[15]

Equally important, social media trivializes the concept of what friendship is. Are you someone's friend because you share information on some newsfeed, timeline, or whatever the latest comment page is called? Would or even *should* you share private information on a site like Facebook? Probably not. Forty-nine percent of adults who use social media report mean or cruel behavior by others. You can only imagine that magnified with preteens and teens who lack maturity that comes with age. Save your personal and important exchanges for face-to-face, or at least live phone, exchanges. Why expose yourself to anything less with true friends?

"The effects of technology on relationships varies from person to person. The way I see it, when communicating online things can get misinterpreted. People seem braver because they are not talking person-to-person, which is more intimate and accurate than online. For example, sarcasm cannot be conveyed in text messages, and the other person could be offended.

"I don't think relationships with people are as strong online as personally. Technology causes a gap in relationships. When I go on Facebook or other social networks and look at friends, I think, I really don't know these people. I look at the news feed and only talked with them once or twice. I don't want to know the details of their lives."— Lucy, high school junior, on technology and friends[9]

Online Privacy

A good way to look at personal exchanges, buying items, and researching online is to assume you have no privacy. Any hacker anywhere in the world can swoop onto a website and steal your information. Companies pay servers to discover what products you prefer. Perverts comb through biographies and ogle over your posted pictures and those of your friends. Parents, school administrators, and police can access certain sites to make sure you are obeying rules and laws. Now future employers check social media to see what you are like and the kind of activities you join. With free speech comes free judgment, so you need to be cautious of what you post.

Of course, you want to allow responsible adults in your life to monitor your exchanges. That's one way to ensure an element of protection. But you may want to keep some communications private. What can you do to keep personal information and thoughts private?

- Only buy products and services from websites that show either *https:* or a yellow padlock on the page that requests information such as credit card numbers or banking figures. These markers indicate that enough information has been scrambled that middle-level snoops cannot access private communications. Although not foolproof, these symbols indicate that the site provides an extra level of security for any sensitive transactions, such as those from vendors, banks, and other sites, that require you to sign up to participate.
- Never list your birth year with the month and date of birth. A hacker who has your complete birthday can match that with a social security number or other information to confirm and steal your identity. Same with addresses (even just street or town names), license plate number, and social security number. Anyone can match a last name with a town or street name and come calling, digitally or personally, whether invited or not.
- Use privacy settings on Facebook and other social media sites, especially if you are not a big fan of other people seeing information posted about your life. Privacy settings limit prying eyes. Only people you prefer to chat or share information with will be allowed access to your pages. If you cannot locate or change the settings, ask a tech-savvy friend or adult for help. It's that important!
- Never post anything on any site that will embarrass you now or in the future. That includes pictures, videos, personal statistics, and gossip about other people.
- Beware: Someone can photograph print conversations, such as texts or e-mails, to keep for later to share with someone who you did not expect to

see them. Even with the simplest recent cell phones, photographers can make copies of your photographs, too. So you need to keep the extreme partying shots to yourself. And never, ever send a nude photo of yourself or any body parts. These communications can come back to haunt you— big time.

- Install a protective program on your computer to block viruses, malware, and other ways of hacking, destroying, or stealing information. Some cost money, but others are free. It's worth investigating. Any time spent on the effort will save hours and considerable stress in the long run, should you get hacked, bullied, or have identity stolen.

- Stop sending chain letters. Besides cluttering everyone else's digital gadgets, they usually infect computers, add cookies (bad tracking stuff), and leave everyone involved open to viruses and other spam.

- Keep passwords to yourself. No one except parents or guardians is entitled to know your business, and that includes access codes. If you think someone else should be able to access your phone or computer, ask a parent or other trusted adult first.

Cyberbullying

Protecting your privacy may be possible. But your image may be harder to guard. As if being bullied to your face isn't bad enough, now teens have to worry about being bullied online. Any bullying is traumatic and terrible. But online bullying has the potential to reach much further than a hallway or playground assault and affect way more people.

A major negative with technology is communicating nasty or untrue messages or photos—altered or not—about you. This negative behavior is called *cyberbullying*. According to the National Bullying Prevention Center, one in every three students will experience bullying this year, and that includes cyberbullying.[16]

What does this involve? Cyberbullying refers to offensive actions intended to hurt someone that come from computers, cell phones, and any other electronic device. The unwanted communication can occur in school or off campus, such as at home or another location. Either way, the behavior disrupts education, so it becomes a serious school problem.

How can you reduce chances of being bullied online? One way is to make sure your school has a clear and thorough policy that protects students from all forms of harassment, including electronic bullying. The statement should define what behaviors constitute a problem. It should cover steps students should take when they feel threatened online. The policy should further spell out exactly what happens to any bully who crosses the line on technology or any other way. The people who contribute to harassment need to be disciplined. Zero tolerance is the best way to send a message that your school community will not tolerate bullies.

The Cyberbullying Research Center recommends a range of discipline for students who bully. The baseline is informing parents. Depending upon the severity of bullying, schools could mandate behavior contracts, loss of privileges, administrative oversight of the students, interventions by guidance counselors, advisers, or social workers, removing the student from class, or enforcing loss of bus privileges. In the worst cases, offending students could be given detention, suspended or expelled, or referred to legal authorities.[17]

Breakups Happen: Sexting Can Last Forever

Casey and Jordan had been dating for a couple months. They decided to see each other exclusively. In fact, they decided to see each other vividly by sexting. They photographed suggestive poses. They shot pictures of themselves in intimate clothing. They e-mailed each other photos of body parts. After about six months, they broke up. Casey deleted photos of Jordan. But Jordan thought it would be cute to keep Casey's images. Casey was offended—and scared.

Since both were underage, technically these pictures were child porn. Some states enacted sexting laws with severe consequences for underage kiddie porn offenders. What does this mean for those of you who think sexting would be fun or an adventure? Don't do it! Resist any pressure to sext.

You cannot be sure how long someone will keep your images. You don't know if you will even stay friends with this person. You cannot control where someone sends your sext. And you haven't a clue when these images might come back to haunt you months and years later. Once an image leaves your camera, it is almost impossible to track and get back.

A Thin Line, MTV's cyberbullying and dating abuse campaign, suggests you ask yourself these questions before you sext:[h]

- Whose idea was this? According to their research, 61 percent of people who sent a sext had been pressured to take the images. If you feel embarrassed and realize sexting has consequences you cannot predict, just say no. It's much better to be called uncool for a short time than suffer later and for an unlimited time, if the pictures wind up posted around school.

- Where will the picture wind up? If you think the images have any chance of reaching an unintended inbox or phone, find something else to share.
- What are the circumstances around taking this picture? Drunken stupor? Party? Being coerced by a date or group of friends? Snapping someone with or without consent? The person in the photo may not want to send embarrassing images. Better to delete instead.
- What image are you trying to communicate? If you think being a sexpot is cool for hooking up with a partner, sexting might work. But how would you feel if friends, parents, teachers, or employers saw these photos? Not so cool now.

Technology and Paying Attention

Television blaring, music in the ears, writing a term paper online, checking text messages, and cell phone bleeps. No problem; some teens can do it all and at the same time. But can they really?

Many believe that technology has created a world that is way too distracting. Even television newscasts show a main reporter bellowing; a written message, sometimes about a different topic, crawling along the bottom of the screen; and another celebrity in a box—all on one screen at the same time.

Where Is a Viewer Supposed To Focus?

This continual bombardment has created younger generations of people—including you—who only know speedy responses and fast-paced presentations. The constant need for instant responses has been called a "distraction addiction."[18] Additionally, teens today are part of a generation with a short attention span for anything. One-third find conventional television so boring they check other technology while watching.[19] Many listen to half messages from parents, then say, "Yeh, yeh, yeh." With teachers, they hear half a lecture before tuning out. The rest sounds like "blah, blah, blah."

Scary Study

Tuning into devices does not automatically mean you will have problems in other aspects of your life. But research shows that those who overdo time online or with cell phones may be in more trouble than those who limit technology.

Investigators at Case Western Reserve University studied 4,000 students from twenty different Ohio high schools. They looked at behaviors of students who texted and accessed social media sites the most. They discovered that about 20 percent of students send more than 120 text messages a day and 10 percent stayed more than three hours a day on social media sites. Another 4 percent participated in both excessive activities. Results revealed that those who used technology the most were at greater risk of participating in dangerous behaviors, such as eating disorders, alcohol and drug abuse, depression, smoking, and sleeping in or cutting classes. The 4 percent who reported greater addiction to technology had double the risk of nonusers for extreme behaviors, such as binge drinking, suicidal thoughts, and fighting.[i]

Technology as an Educational Tool

When technology first appeared, the educational community embraced it as a motivational teaching tool. Computer learning grabbed the attention of students who never liked school. Over time, however, teachers began to question whether technology helped or hindered learning. In the end, it's another mixed bag.

Educators say this generation spends less time reading because an old-fashioned book with rows of words cannot compete with fast-paced visuals and talking images, especially on video games. Additional information is often a click away embedded in the e-book copy, sending the reader in another direction and off topic. Many who do read grumble because they believe reading independently isolates them from online friends. Teens are not used to uninterrupted solitude, and many cannot figure out how to spend time without turning to devices. Others forget how reading expands language and the world, not to mention helps with achieving better grades.

Teachers complain that the more students use mobile phones for texting, for example, the worse offline spelling and punctuation has become. Because teens expect quick responses to problems, this generation tends to check GPS systems, rather than maps. Most have never learned to read a map.

Similarly, math problems are figured out on computer or smartphone calculator, rather than solved by understanding mathematical processes. Simple math is becoming extinct. Salespeople in stores cannot give change without punching in sales because they never mastered the simple addition and subtraction involved. Why bother when a digitally programmed cash register can do the job? Electronic calculators in phones, watches, music players, and calculators diminish the ability to learn basic math skills.

A 2013 Duke University study of computer use among a half-million elementary and junior high students in North Carolina found that "increased high-speed internet access at home was associated with significant declines in math and reading."[20] The latest question becomes, are teens really getting smarter from technology and the overload of information it provides, or are teens losing key skills needed to get through life? Is the Internet affecting how teens think for the better—or dumbing them down?

Myth of Multitasking

Studies indicate that adults over forty have more difficulty with multitasking—and multifocusing—than younger people raised on handling several bits of information, devices, or projects at once. That's the good news for teens. The problem is research refuses to confirm that teens *can* handle many challenges effectively at the same time. Something has to give. Usually that something is time and quality.

Several brain scientists discovered that switching between activities actually takes more time to complete each. The shift requires time before brains adapt to the second task. Researchers at the University of Michigan studied brain effectiveness with volunteer students. Results showed that when "switching back and forth between two tasks, like answering e-mail while writing a paper, brain efficiency decreased by as much as 50 percent, compared with separately completing one task before starting another one."[21]

Scientists at the University of California found similar results from their study of high-tech office workers. They determined that each worker averaged eleven minutes per project. But workers who allowed interruptions or distractions took twenty-five minutes, counting time to readjust and return to their original task.[22] Both studies concluded that the brain works better and quicker on a single task at a time than it does when multitasking, no matter what teens—or their parents—think.

Scientists did report that certain combinations of tasks improved production. Music seems to help cognitive abilities for some people. The right kind of music helps surgeons perform stressful tasks more accurately. Manual laborers work quicker and more precisely with music backgrounds. The thinking is music and manual tasks originate in different parts of the brain, so they do not compete. But research raises questions about music someone dislikes. Distasteful music distracts and reduces productivity. So you need to carefully choose what you listen to while completing important work, like homework.

Technology and Writing and Reading Styles

Texting and e-mailing are quick activities. Messages are to the point. No frills and long explanations. Texting particularly cannot help but leave its mark on writing skills. Similarly, Internet by its sense of immediacy influences reading style.

Teens often respond as soon as they read a message—in a similar no-frills way. Therefore, many teenagers are getting used to fast-paced reading activities. Everything feels urgent, and they don't want to miss anything. So they constantly check their devices. How many times do you see people checking their smartphone while driving (definitely a no-no), riding a bicycle (not great for safety either), or pushing a baby buggy down the street (terrible for a child learning language and connecting with parents)? You might have seen someone texting while doing more than one of these activities at once.

Teens have the mistaken idea they can do everything at once—and do it now. That contrasts with reading books, where characters and stories develop at a slower, more measured rate. Then the question arises, do you still find joy in curling up with a book for recreational reading if you can get instant gratification from a text or an online search? Will you seek out books and longer treatises to discover facts for reports, if you can get something online quickly?

Buyer Beware!

Not all communication is what it seems. Take research for this book, for instance. I tried desperately to find books and online resources to help readers learn more about the topics covered that might relate to their daily communication lives. Indeed, I found several titles and authors. But when I investigated further for professional credentials of the writers and comments or reviews, I found most materials to be self-published. This does not mean that all self-published books lack credibility and aren't worthwhile. But researchers should question literature without any reviews or indications of quality, accuracy, grammar, and writing.

When books, articles, or other written materials go through the usual publishing channels, they have editors who check writing and grammar. Publishers usually send the content to professionals who check facts for accuracy. Stories in these publications are more likely—although not always—true and interesting. With self-published materials, there are no checks. Only one pair of eyes sees the writing, and that's the person who has the most invested in the content reaching publication, the author. Researchers are asked to believe the one person who published the material, no matter how biased or untrue or grammatically incorrect.

Same thing with blogs and social network pages for goods and services. These often pop up first when researching a topic, whether for health care or other classroom topics. But not all websites are created equal. Many webmasters pay search engines, like Google, for more visible placement when someone searches certain words or phrases. What used to be the most reputable site for a topic often gets replaced by the trickiest webmaster who pays the most.

Same with *Wikipedia*, the public encyclopedia-type website. Too often researchers quote *Wikipedia* as gospel. But it can be written and edited by anyone at any time. If readers disagree with the slant and content of an entry, they merely change it. So noting it as a scholarly resource is a mistake. That said, accessing resources at the end of a *Wikipedia* article may be a good way to find additional, more credible resources. If an article displays no resources, be cautious about using the information unless you can confirm it elsewhere.

How to Find Credible Information

Websites run by government, universities, or national professional organizations provide information that comes from experts in the field they cover. That's not to say all private postings and blogs are not valuable in some way. It just tells you to be critical and careful about what and who you note as expert advice. Sometimes, acquiring Internet information—or misinformation—is like going to a fortune teller. What's a novice to do?

- Stick to websites hosted by local and federal governments, professional organizations, colleges, hospitals, museums, historical sites, zoos, and public and university libraries whenever possible. These are monitored and won't get you spammed or otherwise targeted for cookies and other terrible stuff that harms your computer. Few other websites are monitored, which means it might be difficult for you to tell what's true and what isn't.

- Stay away from any website that focuses on one product and tries to sell that product as the answer to your problems.
- Watch out for sites that quickly flip to other sites, rather than allow reading of the page accessed.
- Check out whether something is true or false by going to Snopes.com (or other verifying sites) and inputting the topic. The site alerts readers about hoaxes that might appear via computer. Never believe everything you read online.
- Locate citations on the bottom of the website to see who actually runs the blog/website. Sometimes, you think you are getting unbiased expert information only to find the real site manager has a definite slant about the topic, however subtle.
- Look for more than one source to verify information. Sometimes, when you explore a topic further, you find one source disqualifies the other and relates good reasons why. Many published authors try to find at least three sources before taking something as fact.
- Get a library card. Many libraries now allow users to access valuable search engines from home with the appropriate code on your card. These contain credible information not available through the usual search engines. In fact, whenever you are stumped or want to know how to begin an investigation, ask your local librarian for assistance.
- Never copy information as your own, especially for school papers. All writers deserve to be credited, even those who post online. Your teacher wants to see your work, not ideas and writing from someone else. Viewing several sites and looking at more than one book or article allows you to summarize in your own words without plagiarizing, which you never want to do. That's the same as stealing. Too often teens think the Internet is a cheating tool, meant for copying information without penalty. Don't be fooled.

Communicating between Two Worlds: Then and Now

Just a decade ago, moving to the United States meant barely communicating with loved ones back home. Many foreign communities had no telephone service. Transatlantic, or overseas, phone calls didn't begin until 1927. Calls were so expensive at that time that they were out of reach for most people. An average overseas call back then cost a whopping $200 in today's currency.

Internet connections were unheard of in rural areas. Even snail mail could take a week or two or more to reach its destination. Letters, the main bond between faraway loved ones, often crossed each other before arriving. This gave exchanges a surreal or jerky feeling. One person answered a question another person asked weeks earlier. But senders forgot because they sent other letters with different questions and news. Frustrating.

Recent technology has changed all that. Fiber-optic cables have revolutionized long-distance calling, making calls cheaper and faster. Small communities now have direct phone service. A three-minute call to India that once cost $15 now costs pennies. The cost of calls to the Dominican Republic dropped from $10.59 in 1965 to two cents—or lower—today.[j] And now anyone can purchase a limited use calling card or pay less per call with a monthly unlimited overseas call pack.

Add computers and dirt cheap cell phone packages. Don't forget Skype and similar communication programs that permit calls through computer terminals, some with the ability to see the other person. Immigrants can contact someone back home through Internet. They can continent or country hop within hours. While there are still remote regions of the world, fewer exist each year.[j]

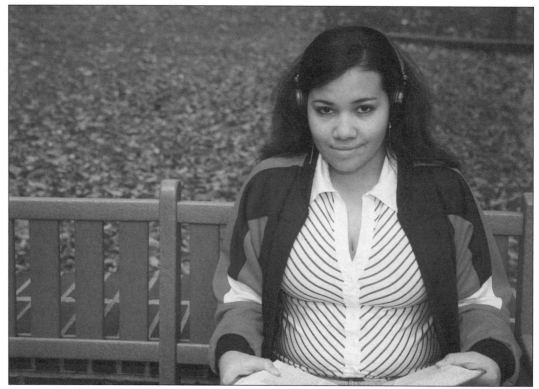

Headsets, earbuds, any device constantly in or on the ears can cause tinnitus or loss of hearing.

You Don't Have to Shout!

A major drawback from some technology is its effect on hearing. There's a fine line between technology that helps teens communicate and high-tech devices that send loud sounds directly into ears (see also chapter 5).

A recent study evaluated two groups of people with hearing tests and surveys of their cell phone habits. One group had tinnitus, ringing in the ear that reduces the ability to hear others speak. Tinnitus can be extremely irritating, affecting how teens focus on what they are doing. The other study group said they did not experience tinnitus. Results indicated that those who used their cell phones at least ten minutes a day had a 71 percent greater risk of tinnitus. Risk levels doubled for those who had talked via cell phone for at least four years.[23]

Researchers figured that microwave exposure from cell phones might be the culprit, damaging the auditory pathway. Although more research is needed, researchers suggest limiting this kind of noise exposure. Hold shorter conversations. Text. Or try a hands-free device or landline, especially for long calls. The farther the phone is from your head, the less your ears will be affected.

Malarie's Story

For years everyone told Malarie to stop using a hand-held hair dryer. Her mother said it was too noisy. Her father warned her about hearing loss. Her brother, well, he was generally annoying, so anything he said about hair dryers didn't count. Malarie insisted she could only use a hair dryer with the brush to straighten her hair. And the only way to dry her hair the way she wanted was with the hand-held kind. She was sure the cautions didn't apply to her. Her hearing was sound and would continue that way forever.

As the years passed, her ears would suddenly plug and unplug. From time to time she felt fluttering in her ears. Ringing came and went, alternating between ears. On two occasions, she suddenly lost hearing completely in one ear. Yet, she kept drying her hair with the noisy hand-held dryer—daily.

An audiologist claimed the fluttering was probably from allergies and fluid in the middle ear. But she said the other three symptoms could have come from sound buildup after so many years using the hair dryer. Hair dryers give off the same decibels, seventy, as lawn mowers, only they are used closer to the head. Some technology can actually be harmful.[k]

Social Media and the Greater World

It's official! Many perspective employers and high school and college administrators want to know which social media you use. Partly, this is to consider how tech-savvy you might be, a bonus to their company or business or to completing reports. But they may also be interested in the image you present online.

School administrators may peek at social media. Maybe they want to know who your friends are, if a problem arises. Or they want to know if you posted—or bragged—about getting into mischief, such as getting answers to a test or pulling a prank on another student in school.

What message does this have for you now and in the future? Remember to think before you post. Be cautious about what you choose to share, whether personal information about you and your friends and family or pictures.

One way to decide what to share is to consider whether you would like the topic to come up during a job interview or meeting with a school adviser or principal. Of course, you have free speech and can post what you want, depending on

Break the Technology Habit

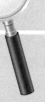

What do you do with your seeming addiction to technology? Several authors have written tomes about just that topic—and more are sure to come. Here are some suggestions they offer:

- Take a technology holiday. Start with a few hours unconnected. Or consider unplugging during certain activities, such as outings with friends or family dinners. Gradually build up the time not checking e-mail and social media.
- Be mindful of time spent offline. Step back from the computer and smartphone. Meditate or take deep breaths, both ideas to reduce stress and recharge overwhelmed brains.
- Evaluate the time spent on each digital activity. Eliminate the activities/ sites that take up the most time.
- Turn off cells during class. Your grades may depend on it. One study put text messaging during class at 58 percent of students.[1] You are smarter than that.
- Make driving a tech-free activity. Many lives depend on the ability to focus.
- Tell friends you will not answer their tweets or e-mails during certain hours.
- Find new hobbies, activities, and chores you have always wanted to explore or accomplish.
- Make plans to meet friends in person for an activity. Set ground rules, so everyone knows this activity will be digital free.
- Schedule e-mail sessions. Maybe you won't feel so addicted if you know you have a special time to read and respond.
- Prepare a topic to talk about, if you and your friends find face-to-face initial communicating difficult. At first, it might feel awkward, but you need to put substance back into your communications, something that might have been lost in the speedy, high-tech world of communicating in tweets, instant messages, and social media sites.

house rules. But that right extends to the freedom of a potential college intake administrator or potential employer to make judgments based on the sensitive posting.

Resources

Organizations/Websites

Alliance for Technology Access
1119 Old Humboldt Road
Jackson, TN 38305
731-554-5282 (voice); 731-554-5284 (TTY)
ataccess.org
National organization that provides referrals, advocacy, and information to help increase the use of technology by anyone with disabilities or functional limitations to help them participate more fuly in their community.

Cyberbullying Research Center
www.cyberbullying.us
According to the center, this online website "serves as a clearinghouse of information concerning the ways adolescents use and misuse technology." The site offers resources and research for students, parents, and school personnel about ways to prevent and deal with cyberbullying.

Teenangels
www.teenangels.org
This division of WiredSafety is run by thirteen- to eighteen-year-old volunteers. They are specially trained to talk with younger kids and other teens about safe online surfing.

WiredSafety
www.wiredsafety.org
World's largest online safety, education, and help group for cyberspace users. Volunteers from ages seven to ninety-six help and support victims of cybercrimes and harassment, assist with law enforcement, and educate teens and parents about safe and responsible Internet usage.

Yoursphere Media Foundation and Coalition for Internet Safety Education and Reform
"I Choose" Anti-Bullying Campaign

www.whatdoyouchoose.org
Powered by YourSphere.com, this social network has been created "by kids and teens for kids and teens" to respect and encourage positive online interactions.

Books: Nonfiction

Fleischmann, Carly, and Arthur Fleischmann. *Carly's Voice: Breaking through Autism.* New York: Simon & Schuster, 2012. Firsthand computer exchange between a teen with autism and her father that discusses what her life with autism has been like.

Steiner-Adair, Catherine. *The Big Disconnect: Protecting Childhood and Family Relationships in the Digital Age.* New York: HarperCollins, 2013. Written for adults, but this book is for everyone who values family and friendships in the computer era. Text has plenty of examples that will hit home for preteens and teens.

Video

"I Forgot My Phone"
Charlene deGuzman, writer, actor
Miles Crawford, director
www.youtube.com/watch?v=OINa46HeWg8
Two-minute video that documents a woman going through her day and experiencing how individuals are so involved in their technology that they are missing the moments they are trying to document.

LOOKING AHEAD: BOOSTING COMMUNICATIONS SKILLS ALL AROUND

No matter what type of speech and language challenge teens have, there are always ways to improve communications. Sure a speech problem can be frustrating. Remember how annoying those people are who think their saying "Slow down" or "Relax" will magically make words come easier? What about others who avoid eye contact when you talk too slowly or cannot find the correct words to say? Or those who won't recognize that your problems may be lifelong and not your fault?

Even with these outside influences trying to fight progress, there are always options to make your communication life easier. The best way to begin improving is to take stock of how you communicate with others. Ask yourself the following questions:

- Do you find others looking at you strangely when you speak?
- Are you often misunderstood or do you get unexpected responses?
- How can you improve interactions at home and within the community?
- What type of image would you like to project?
- What are ways you can reach this image goal?

Honestly evaluate specific changes that would improve your day-to-day activities. Then decide whether any of the following suggestions hit home.

Communicating with Others

A sign of solid relationships is feeling comfortable enough to tell others how to help you better. You may be one of those teens who views asking for what you

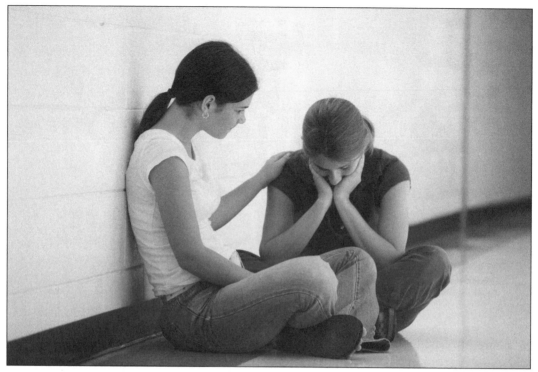

Talking with a trusted friend relieves stress and may help with a troublesome situation.

need as a sign of weakness. But it's not weakness to ask for assistance, especially when communication challenges are involved. If those close to you cannot be helpful, perhaps you need to find objective outside assistance. Consider a speech pathologist, social worker, psychologist, guidance counselor, other responsible adult, or tutor or mentor of any age.

If you already see a professional and not much is clicking for you, trust your judgment. Find a different person. In the meantime, consider the following ideas to help improve your life overall.

Listening: The Ultimate Communication Weapon

No information about communication—speech and language—would be complete without emphasis on the importance of listening. This is the process of receiving spoken messages, and experts view the skill as part of the circle of life for successful conversations. Why is listening so important? Listening is how you obtain meaning from what others say. Without active listening, you cannot respond in an appropriate fashion. That is true with friends, with family, and in school, or at work. As the old Turkish proverb says, "If speaking is silver, then listening is gold."

Listening–All the Way to the Supreme Court

Supreme Court justice Sonia Sotomayor admits in her autobiography that she was never shy about speaking her mind. But she credits much of her success as a student, lawyer, and eventual judge to her ability to listen.

"Listening was second nature to me," she writes. "My friends confided in me, unloaded their problems, and leaned on me for advice. . . . When I was little, listening and watching for cues had seemed like the key to survival in a precarious [shaky, dangerous] world. I notice when people hesitate or get defensive, when they care more about what they're saying than they'll admit, or when they're too quick about brushing something off. So much is communicated in tone of voice, in subtleties of expression, and in body language."[a]

People listen to others for a variety of reasons. Some merely want to understand what someone is saying. The best way to know what beliefs someone is advocating is to listen. Do you agree or disagree with these beliefs? The only way to decide for sure is to listen.

Others are trying to bolster a relationship. Or they want specific directions, such as in class. How else can you discover what critical information goes into reports and tests? How else can you decide how to answer questions in class or on the job? How else will you discover where to meet friends in the cafeteria after the bell rings?

Listening is one of the key tools in your communication toolbox. Many educators believe that active listening—when you really engage in what someone else is saying—is more essential than speaking in the communication exchange. Research agrees. According to one survey, listening takes up an average of 55 percent of daily communications. Speaking involves half of that at 23 percent, reading takes up 13 percent, and writing engages 9 percent.[1] No matter what the speech and language challenges, everyone can improve communications—and relationships—by improving listening skills.

Roadblocks to Effective Listening

Do you find yourself unconsciously or consciously putting up barriers to listening? Your body sits in class, but your mind goes out to lunch. All you hear the teacher saying is "blah, blah, blah." Probably at one time or another most people have participated in this kind of nonlistening.

Cultural Differences in Listening

In some families, everyone talking at once is the only way to survive. Ever watch *The View* on television? Panel members may try to listen to each other, but often viewers think the panel could benefit from a referee. Guests on the infamous interview couch surrounded by chattering panelists frequently comment about their inability to get in a word—and to feeling overwhelmed when more than one person speaks at once.

Not so in some Native American communities. Keen listening has been a skill nurtured from early childhood and valued throughout maturity. Since Native American culture used to pass from one generation to another orally, each word counted. Elders emphasized storytelling as a way to teach community history and life lessons. Without good listening skills, transmitting culture would never occur.

The reasons for zoning out are legion. Educators and corporate trainers who study this sort of behavior have pinpointed several common barriers to productive listening:[2]

- Lack of interest. Maybe the topic isn't your thing. Or information doesn't jibe with your needs. But you can't leave, especially if you are in class or on the job. You need to overcome your disinterest and deal with it. Not always easy.
- Negative reaction to the speaker. Perhaps you never liked the speaker personally, so you tend to dismiss whatever this person says. You find voice quality or other mannerisms offensive. You cannot stand the person's attitude. Even the speaker's clothes appear distracting. This is another problem to work on moving past.
- Daydreaming. How many times have you spaced out during a presentation? You stare out the window, wishing you were somewhere else. Or your mind has sailed to other places: A fight with your parents. Thoughts of a weekend date with a special person. Worry of an upcoming test or important game. If your mind is elsewhere, you usually have trouble crafting responses to questions or following directions, such as in class.

Take notes or hold something, and not a cell phone, to help you stay focused.

- Mentally battling the speaker. In this situation, there is probably nothing the speaker says after a certain point that you find agreeable. If there is, you will never know because your mind already grabbed onto a word or phrase, and you go off mentally arguing with the speaker. You miss key points. You distort what the speaker says. You need to hear the speaker out and try to stay objective.

- Bad attitude. Maybe the negative reaction is your attitude. Perhaps you are a half-empty kind of person who sees the negative in anything anyone says. Time to turn around this thinking, especially if you want or need information from the speaker.

    One way to turn around a negative brain is to start a gratitude journal. Seriously. Try to write something positive about each day. You could write about a pleasant encounter with friends, how you bravely raised your hand in class, or how you finally crawled out of bed in time for school. Soon one positive observation turns into more than one each day, and you grow into a positive person. Sounds hokey, but it works.

- Need to talk. Some people feel whatever they have to say is more important than waiting their turn to respond. They become so focused on their talking that they miss the gist of a conversation. These same people interrupt, and in some cases disrupt, a presentation, including in concerts or theater. They are insensitive to others who want to listen. In most circles, this is simply bad manners. You cannot talk and listen at the same time. Won't work.

- Attention-deficit/hyperactivity disorder (ADHD). Maybe you have a condition, such as ADHD, that prevents you from sitting still enough to focus. Everything but the speaker attracts your attention. Your mind swirls with overstimulation that prevents constructive listening. You notice every speck on the floor or each mark on the bulletin board. Some teachers provide corrals, mini desk enclosures, to block out excess stimulation. Or you could take notes or perform some other activity that is absorbing but still allows you to listen. If these suggestions don't prove workable, check with a therapist or doctor about behavior treatments or medication that can help calm you enough to listen.

Overcoming Barriers to Listening

You can always become a better listener, even if you truly believe you attend to others when they speak. But developing better listening skills requires practice

Mayoral Candidates and Poor Listening Skills

Lack of attention plus hardcore mobile device overusage appeared front and center, as on the front page of the *New York Times*. A reporter called out politician behavior during a forum for the New York 2013 race for mayor. He saw one candidate sending cell phone messages, while another monitored *two* devices at once. A third texted with his daughter, and a fourth checked Twitter and Facebook accounts—compulsively. And this was while they were supposed to be listening to each other and audience questions.

Candidates appeared bored, uninterested, and totally disconnected from voters, who have a right to expect better behavior. After the bad behavior was revealed, advisers tried to cover for their bosses. One said he knew candidates should never look distracted. But he also knew in this fast-paced communication era people wanted instant answers to questions.

Still, this adviser now counsels candidates with the usual advice, plus one extra tip: "If you are on TV, wear blue. Sit on your suit jacket. Don't swivel in your chair. Don't click your pen." And now: "Don't check your emails."[b]

and conscious commitment, especially when a communication disorder is involved.

Whether in general conversation or the classroom, the best way to show you are engaged is to establish eye contact with the speaker. Your body should be welcoming, as in relaxed, and show you are involved in the interaction. Sit tall, if in a chair. Relax your arms and legs, although not sprawling over furniture. If possible lean toward the speaker, rather than taking on a "show me" challenging posture. Focus on the speaker and the message being said. Eliminate distracting pens, cell phones, and anything that encourages fidgeting. Your undivided attention sends a powerful message that the speaker is worth listening to and important to you.

Rapt attention is not enough, though. You need to concentrate and keep your mouth shut until someone finishes talking. Never interrupt as the person goes along. This includes refraining from finishing sentences. Keeping quiet can be tough when you want to speed up a glacially moving conversation or when you know what the person might say. Similarly, never put words in someone else's

> **❗ Listen the Native American Way**
>
> ◉ Remember to listen in the traditional Native America way mentioned in chapter 7. Only the person who holds the stick is allowed to speak. Others must listen respectfully. After each person has spoken, the group crafts decisions together from the different points of view. Can't get much better listening than that.[c]

mouth. Even speakers you dislike are entitled to their own thoughts and opinions. Never assume you know everything. As religion professor Howard Hendricks is credited with saying, "The principle of listening is to develop a big ear rather than a big mouth."[3]

One of the most difficult aspects of conversing, if you like to interrupt, is to hold arguments until the other person finishes speaking. A good way to keep your cool is to take notes. Once the points are on paper or in the computer, you will be sure not to forget them. Then you can refocus on the speaker and the rest of the conversation or presentation. You may have seen presidential candidates in a debate taking notes.

Thinking—and Communicating—Positively

Listen for items in the message where you find agreement. This keeps you more positive and engaged until the end of the message. Far better than finding fault and jumping to conclusions, which turns off listeners. Once you take a negative mind-set, you don't hear what someone is saying. You think you know it all already—which you don't.

> **Speech Anxiety**
>
> Nervous about public speaking? You are definitely not alone. While fear of public speaking hits some harder than others, studies show that about 75 percent of people admit to anxiety at the thought of talking in front of anyone let alone large groups.

"It is even scarier than rattlesnakes," says Paul Witt, assistant professor of communications at Texas Christian University. "The idea of making a presentation in public is the number one fear reported by people in the United States."[d]

The good news is once someone starts a presentation, the fear usually recedes. And there are things you can do to ease the concern. Dr. Witt and others have several suggestions for anxiety symptoms.

Decide if you are the kind of person who speaks more easily on a full or empty stomach. Perhaps something in the middle would work best. Eat a small but healthy snack to keep your stomach from growling or distracting you because of hunger. But don't eat enough to result in gas or the need to race to the bathroom, which is a good thing to do *before* presenting. Speaking of preparing the body, be sure to get a good night's sleep before presentation day. Sleeping restores the mind, helps your memory, and keeps you awake and better able to cope during the presentation.[e]

Dry mouth from anxiety? Sip water, and keep a glass handy in case you get dry mouth during the speech, something even pros experience. Knees knock? Shift your weight and flex your knees, or move a few feet at a time, like you are strolling. And remember to look at the audience as you speak.

What to do with your hands? That can be more complicated, depending upon whether or not you are from a culture that values talking with your hands. If you are not gesturing, put your hands down at your side. This looks more natural. To stop hands from trembling either clasp them together or hold notes or a podium or stand. Holding something serves two purposes at once. Besides stopping jittery hands, leaning in, such as on the podium and toward the audience, sends a sturdier, more committed message about you and what you are saying.

Similarly, know where to look during the speech. Look at the person in the back of the audience. That way, everyone in between you and the last row will believe you are looking at them. As you become more comfortable while speaking, try to look at different sections of the last row.

Voice quivering? Remember to take a deep breath or two before starting. Breathing deeply transports much-needed oxygen to the brain. This will help you calm down and think clearly. If you find yourself nervous during the speech, take another breath. And you don't have to shout to be heard. While you don't want to

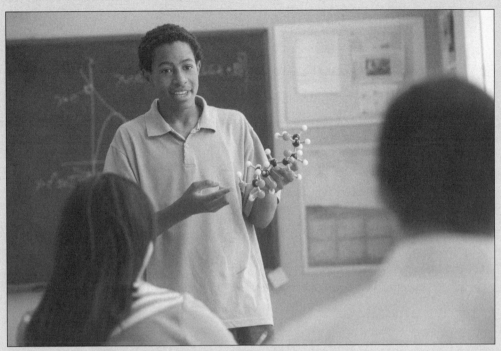

Presenting to the class takes planning, practice—and confidence.

mumble, research shows that a quieter voice forces the audience to listen better. This is especially true if you have a microphone. Leave yelling into a microphone to punk rockers.

Remember to smile at the audience. Smiling is a real crowd-pleaser. A smile puts everyone at ease, including you. Dr. Witt also recommends ignoring perspiration. Everyone else does.

The last point is probably the most important. The best way to reduce anxiety and build confidence is to practice before giving a presentation. Practice voice inflection and gestures that help emphasize main points. Run through visuals you intend to use, so you feel comfortable accessing them. Keep visuals simple and use them as a guide, like a prompt or outline. Never fill the slides with text and read from them. Boring!

Practicing in front of a mirror or recording the presentation is a good beginning. Best to grab a friend, sibling, or parent to listen to your presentation. Objective observers can offer meaningful feedback, such as good advice about how to look more natural, smile more, or gesture less or more. Remember that a little fear motivates. The rest you can work with and overcome.

"I recently found myself in a phone conversation with a professor of my university that I had never met before. We chatted for some time while I wondered exactly why he had called me, until he got to the point— he needed someone to speak at a benefactor dinner the coming week. Feeling completely confident in my public speaking abilities, I accepted the offer, and at the dinner, my speech ended up being the highlight of the night. I give credit to the fact that I was taught how to properly give a speech and how to deliver it confidently. I've realized more and more that my public speaking skills give me a very noticeable edge above those students who don't possess them, and in a world that is driven by powerfully-spoken people, teaching that skill to students should be on the top of every school's priority list."—Sarah Vans, college student [f]

Tips for Acing High School

Experts list different skills that first-year high schoolers need to succeed by senior year. Each enhances the ability to communicate effectively. If adopted, these actions can help launch you successfully into the world of college and work.

1. Manage Your Time

No surprise here. Without the ability to allot time effectively, you cannot get your work done, study for tests, and engage in social activities, too. But remember that whatever contributes to a speech and language challenge may require extra time to complete this list.

According to FamilyEducation.com, high school students spend an average of thirty-five hours a week in class.[9] By college, however, that number drops to fifteen to eighteen hours of class time. Nonclass hours demand management between effective study and social time. The earlier you learn to manage time wisely the stronger your foundation for handling higher education and a calendar that may also include afterschool activities and employment.

To help plan your time, keep a date book or calendar or daily planner, similar to ones required in various high schools. Some students prefer to document schedules on smart phones. Regularly scheduling daily activities allows you to see if you double-booked, overscheduled, or left too much unproductive free time. Check off each activity after completion. It's rewarding to see a visual account of progress with your accomplishments. Calendars get you in the habit of handling time wisely. In turn, this allows extra time you might need to deal with challenging communication issues.

2. Create Good Study Habits

Study habits vary with the individual. You might write papers easily in the center of a noisy coffee house, while someone else needs total silence to concentrate. Other students line up neat piles of books and papers, while a few might feel more comfortable surrounded by clutter. These and other quirks of studying are important to figure out, again the earlier the better.

The critical point is to carve out time each day for study. Keep to the schedule even if no test or paper is due. Use the time to work ahead, read ahead, or lose yourself in a good book, magazine, or newspaper to catch up on current events.

Maintaining effective study habits allows you to prepare for class and complete assignments on time. Setting aside time gives you an opportunity to schedule assistance, therapy, or tutoring, if necessary. Reading outside assigned projects builds vocabulary and knowledge that helps with communication and learning.

Once you find a place where you like to study, keep a supply of study materials there. By leaving study tools, such as writing implements, paper notebooks, planners, books, and computer, in one place, you save time and energy better used for class and studying.

During study time, review notes from previous classes. Get updates if you notice holes in notes you took. Find a study buddy, if taking notes is difficult for you. Develop a strategy for arranging information once you have taken notes.

Some students use colored index cards or folders with separators labeled with different topics to help them organize. Still have trouble with note taking? Ask the teacher if you can record lessons or use the teacher's notes from the class. Some teachers post outlines online about what they discuss during lectures.

3. Adjust Attitude

Let's face it: studying takes commitment and motivation. Without these, school can be a real drag. To get motivated, set attainable goals and work hard to reach them. Reevaluate goals at regular intervals and set new ones, if priorities change, which they will. Decide that schoolwork comes first. Then refocus, keep a positive attitude, and do your best in school. Remember: No one is good at everything, but everyone can be good at trying.[h]

4. Build Self-Confidence

Ever listen to adults talk about their high school years? To a person, they discuss what low self-esteem they had. That includes people from every clique: jocks, supposedly cool kids, and nerds. The point here is you are not alone. On the positive side, high school shakes up middle school cliques and widens opportunities for new friends and activities. But a larger building and greater number of teens and classes can be scary. Add a communication challenge, and wading through teen years can seem even scarier.

Get involved from the beginning in at least one school activity that seems remotely interesting. Joining something of interest connects you to school in a positive way. An involving activity gives you a common interest and topics to discuss with at least a few other students. You can always drop or add activities as interests change. But you can count on at least one thing to make you feel better about yourself.

Smiling goes a long way toward opening yourself to meeting other students. And meeting people is a real confidence builder. Sounds simple, but it works. Who would you rather approach, someone who looks gruff and walks with shoulders slumped and head down or someone with a sparkly smile who makes eye contact? Smiling is contagious—and in a good way.

5. Prepare for Something New and Exciting

The best way to reduce the anxiety of starting anything new is to plan ahead. Begin by deciding on transportation to the new school *before* the first day of classes. If you need to take the bus, arrange for a bus pass, if that's required, and practice bus trips. Same with practicing routes for bicycling or walking. If you are still not certain, invite someone who knows the route to join you.

Visit the new school before classes start. Locate rooms where your classes will be, and walk through the schedule to plot routes. It's common for students to get lost traveling from class to class. Best to experience the route without students and crowded hallways.

Planning also involves contacting a friend before school starts. Nothing worse than entering a huge cafeteria not knowing anyone or where to sit. Arrange to meet at least one person, so neither of you eat alone.

If you are the kind of person who never seems organized or easy to please when dressing, decide what you want to wear the night before the first day of school. Make sure your favorite outfits are clean and ready to wear. You don't want to miss a ride because nothing looks right. Even if dressing isn't your thing, you will feel more confident wearing clothes that raise your comfort level.

Remember that everyone entering high school—or college—is new to the school. Probably each person has the same reservations as you do. Teens think they invented whatever they are going through, whether or not they have communication challenges.

The good news about your better listening is that you are being a role model. You are modeling behavior you want from others—that they listen to what you say.

Handling Parents

Try to remember that parents usually want the best for their children. But they are often unsure what to do. Part of their misgivings may come from uncertainty about how to act or react in today's fast-paced, high-achieving culture. Partly they may not have figured out how to handle your communication differences.

Maybe they feel guilty, like somehow they caused your speech and language issue. They may show their guilt by being overprotective. Or they may try to correct what you say and how you say it—all the time.

You are old enough to request a little space, within household boundaries of course. See if any of these parental suggestions prove helpful in your situation:

1. Tell parents to take a break from constant correction. Again, parents usually mean well. They might figure if they correct your speech and language—either in how you talk or write or both—that perhaps their corrections will stick, and you will be magically fixed. You may appreciate their homework assistance, within bounds. But constant reminders of how you talk or write only undermine your confidence.

Best to specifically limit the circumstances when corrections will be appreciated, and when they are not. Be respectful but firm when having the conversation. For example, say that you might appreciate edits on a school paper, but no one wants their e-mails or letters sent home from camp corrected for grammar and returned. How demeaning! Similarly, remind parents that finishing sentences or talking for you to others—particularly in your presence—is definitely not cool. Also a self-esteem buster!

2. Request regular family meetings. Many families include members who are overwhelmed with work, school, and activities. They find little time to truly listen to each other. Ask your family to schedule regular meetings at a mutually agreed-upon time when everyone must be present and all parties must turn off electronic devices.

Trouble communicating respectfully? Remember the Native American talking stick (see chapter 7). This is a way to hold nonjudgmental, respectful meetings where each person holding the stick takes a turn talking without interruption. Many families need this sort of structure to connect in a positive way. Perhaps yours does, too.

3. Suggest that parents work with you about bad grades rather than freak out. Make sure your parents know that you feel badly enough about a low grade or test result. If parents want to be productive, they can bolster a positive work environment. They can brainstorm with you ways to improve. If neither of you can come up with suggestions, either you (preferably you speak for yourself first) or a parent contact the teacher for clarification of problems. Review work habits, difficult subject areas, handling homework. Plan together ways to monitor improvement. But let parents know that ultimately school is your responsibility, and you are trying your best.

4. Communicate with your parents. Teens like to be independent of adults. That is normal. You don't have to spill every private thought to your parents. But remember that parents are on your team for important things. They can provide feedback about something bothering you; assistance with school, work, or a relationship problem; need for extra help due to your communication challenges; or help when being bullied. Don't keep secrets that can harm you. Stay connected with trusted adults.

Dating with a Speech and Language Problem

Dating and spending time with a special person is another important right of passage. Having a speech and language disorder does not change this interest. In fact, it points out how similar you are to anyone without a communication problem. Just like other teens, you might be asking yourself if you are ready to handle the pressures and responsibilities of dating.

Parents might solve this dilemma for you by putting a restriction on the age you can begin dating. But the more important sign of readiness is your social age. Are you responsible at home or at school? Do you meet deadlines, know how to interact with others in a positive way, and complete chores?

Look carefully at how your speech and language challenges affect how you function. Do your communication challenges interfere with self-confidence? Or does talking differently bury the real personality inside because you tend to stay in the shadows rather than speak? You need to decide whether you are ready to work around and overcome communication difficulties. Only then can you give to someone else in a relationship.

Here are some important questions to ask yourself, no matter what your communication style:

- Do you engage in risky behavior? If the answer is *yes*, this question might point to low self-esteem. You may be trying to prove something to yourself or get attention by acting in extreme ways that are dangerous, such as with drugs, sex, fast driving, or trick bicycle riding.
- Are you able to interpret social cues that might cause a problem dating? Knowing when to stop talking, when to listen, or when someone is turned off is important to connecting with someone special.
- Do you have problems standing up for yourself? A *yes* response might indicate that you can be a pushover. You will follow peer pressure—even go along with some ideas you know are stupid—or become easily intimidated, or worse, allow yourself to be bullied or pushed into doing something you regret or makes you feel uncomfortable.
- Do you have knowledge of your beliefs and stand by them? You need the confidence to say *no* and mean it in a dating relationship, particularly when the relationship moves to the next level of physical intimacy.
- Do you demand the same respect as anyone else? You may have a communication challenge, but that doesn't mean you don't have the same

On the Job with Dyslexia

Jeremy desperately wanted a job. But he worried that having dyslexia might keep him from finding one. So he brainstormed with his speech therapist about alternatives. He discovered that his problem with reading could be easily solved in the workplace. He could ask someone to read articles to him. He could ask coworkers to leave voice-mail messages instead of sending e-mails. He could record directions, so he could listen to them until he understood what to do. He learned that with a little thought and planning ahead there is always a way to make his choices succeed.[i]

range of feelings as others have. These need to respected, no matter what circumstances arise.

Exciting Interviews

As you mature, you will have opportunities to participate in an interview. Perhaps you are trying out for a group or activity. Or you want a certain job. Or the college you prefer requires a personal interview with the program head. Interviews are a way for someone outside your immediate circle to get to know you and evaluate whether you are a good match for what they have to offer.

No one likes getting sized up. But interviews are part of life. Therefore, use the occasion to shine. Interviews provide an occasion to present your best self. They give you the opportunity to meet new people who are looking at you through the eyes of their specific needs.

Interviews, however, come under the heading of stress producers, much like speaking before groups. If you have a communication challenge, an interview might trigger even more anxiety. You wonder how you can make yourself understood. You worry that you will be judged by a speech issue that is obvious.

The good news in today's high-tech market is that job hunting often begins online, which takes more skill in writing clearly than speaking. If someone is interested in talking with you, often that starts with a phone call. You can ask what will be discussed, so you can plan—and practice—responses before the phone interview. You can ease into the scarier parts of a face-to-face interview one step at a time.

One way to reduce anxiety in any situation is to think of the worst thing that can happen. With an interview, you can get rejected. You can handle that, correct? Like anyone else, you move on to the next interview.

Talia's Story: In Her Own Words

My dad is the kind of guy who never stops harping. When he learned I had a job interview, he pounded home the idea of planning ahead. Hey, I don't know what I want to do five minutes from now. Why should I plan for an interview next week?

To get him off my back, I explored activities about the job I was seeking. As he suggested—or rather ordered me to do—I listed what I could say about myself—both positive and negative. Then I prepared a list of possible interview questions. We practiced together, with him asking the questions and me answering, or trying to. Embarrassing. But I learned I was better on my feet with surprise responses than I thought. I would never tell him, but the practicing helped. I was more confident during the interview, *and* I got the job.[j]

Even with rejection, the interview is still a success. You have met someone new. You have participated in an exchange that is another learning experience that will help you achieve success later. You have a benchmark to compare what worked and what did not work, so you can improve your interview skills. Here are some guidelines to help reduce interview anxiety and increase chances of success:[4]

- Investigate ahead of time what the job or program entails. That way, you can refer to specifics during the conversation and tailor your talents to the needs of the situation. For example, if you are interviewing for a camp counselor position, you can talk about swimming or horseback riding skills or your experience babysitting. Interviewers often want to know why you are interested in their program. They want to know why they should consider you for the position above others. They want to know your strengths and weaknesses and any relevant experience for the post.

  Besides figuring out what you might be asked, prepare questions to ask the interviewer about the job or program. Questions mean you are interested, not that you are not smart enough to hire. You may not be the best talker, but you need to convey that you have the necessary skills—the ability to organize or be friendly or calculate numbers quickly or are creative, whatever the situation requires—that other candidates might not have.
- Role-play an interview. Ask someone to help you in the give-and-take conversation of an interview. This may not come naturally to you, especially with adults. Practicing answers to questions beforehand ensures the responses come out smoothly. Practice different responses to sample questions

you think might arise. Also identify which capabilities you want to insert into responses, such as computer skills or athletic ability. Be serious about the role playing. Look your pretend interviewer in the eye when talking. Employ your best listening skills.

- Bring items that will help you. For example, if you are applying to art school, bring a portfolio of your work. Show anything that will give an interviewer a sense of your capabilities.

- Learn to communicate with adults. Shake those "duhs," "likes," "yahs," and "ya knows" when speaking. Leave the chip on your shoulder at the door, you know, the one that comes naturally because the interviewer is an authority figure. But speak up for yourself, so you don't sound like you have a mouth full of cotton.

- Practice the fine points of communicating in an interview. Greet the interviewer in a friendly manner. If you shake hands, do so with a strong handshake. Sit tall in the chair to look more assertive and attentive. Whatever you are interviewing for be upbeat and enthusiastic.

- Be on time for the interview. Being late causes you more anxiety before the interview even begins. Moreover, tardiness messes up the interviewer's schedule and sends a message that you are irresponsible, which reflects on how capable or interested you might be, whether true or not. Why start off on the interviewer's wrong side before the interview begins? In fact, come early enough for a bathroom trip to check how you look and take a deep calming breath.

- Look your best. Communication involves more than what you say and how you say it. Valid or not, studies show that interviewers make snap judgments during the first five face-to-face minutes. This does not mean dressing like a fashion plate. To make a good impression, make sure you are clean, neat, shaven, and odor free. Comb your hair, and cover any revealing body parts. Looking different or sexy might work in school halls or at the mall, and tattoos and piercings are more common these days. But the reality is, in most interview situations, clean-cut still comes out ahead.

- Discuss special communication issues that might be apparent. Be honest. If you need louder phone devices due to reduced hearing, you should explain that. If stuttering is your challenge, make sure the interviewer knows your other qualities that suit the position you are seeking. Briefly address potential negatives quickly, then move on to your strong points.

- Send a thank-you note. Like everyone, interviewers like to be appreciated for their time and effort. Find a business letter thank you online or purchase a thank-you card. Hard copy is preferable. But if you can only manage an e-thanks, that is better than no thanks.

Communicating on the Job

Only you and your family can decide whether you can handle work and school-work. A communication challenge should not interfere with working any more than for other teens. You just need to be more aware of the type of work you choose. Be realistic if you have certain communication challenges. For example, if you stutter, you may not want a job selling at a store. If you have a learning disability that causes an attention problem, you may need an environment where you can move around, rather than a desk job in a large room with many people at desks.

If you decide to work, think about the type of job and environment that suits your skills and interests. Brainstorm ideas with a trusted adult. Then embark on a job-hunting journey that will take organization and persistence.

Figure out the type of establishment and work tasks you prefer. Tell everyone you know what you prefer. Networking, using contacts who know contacts, is helpful with job hunting. Investigate stores, offices, nonprofit groups, camps, and recreation and community centers near you. Check for jobs on local employment

Test Your Interests: Job Shadowing or Internships

One way to test the job waters is to apply for an internship or a block of time shadowing a professional. An internship is a situation where you offer your time and labor in exchange for on-the-job experience. A professional at a company, business, or nonprofit agrees to supervise you acquiring skills. This situation could be for a limited time or specific number of hours or over the summer or a school break. You could be paid—or not. Either way, you likely would gain invaluable experience, while figuring out if this is an area you would like to pursue.

Shadowing is limited in time, also, perhaps a few hours or a day or two. Only with shadowing you follow professionals through their day as an observer. No labor involved, unless you agree to it. The good thing about shadowing is you discover what someone in that particular job actually does. Armed with this information you can add or subtract it on your to-do list of possible careers or job choices.

websites or in the newspaper. Distribute leaflets throughout the neighborhood that advertise if you want to babysit, pet sit, mow lawns, or perform odd jobs.

A job is a good way to build confidence. Employment gives you organization skills and experience dealing with different kinds and ages of people. Work makes you feel you are like everyone else, with or without a communication challenge.

Know Your Rights to Work: It's the Law

Two major federal laws cover rights for individuals with diverse disabilities, including speech and language impairment. The Rehabilitation Act of 1973 specifically prohibits discrimination in federal agencies or programs that receive federal funding. Section 504 of the act affirms that "no qualified individual with a disability in the United States shall be excluded from, denied the benefits of, or be subjected to discrimination under place of employment"[k] that contracts or requests funding from the government. Accommodations include "effective communication with people who have hearing . . . disabilities." This means you can report any business that either denies service or refuses to hire you because of a communication problem, if you are otherwise competent to handle the job.

Based on civil rights and Rehabilitation Act legislation, the U.S. government created the Americans with Disabilities Act (ADA), last updated in 2010. The ADA is more inclusive than previous laws regarding civil rights of anyone with a disability. This law has been called the "equal opportunity law for people with disabilities."[l] It has a specific section that deals with communication, both as a customer and employee. The law says businesses have a responsibility to provide oral interpreters or sign language for the hearing impaired, if cost does not prove a burden. The law also permits businesses to employ updated technology, such as video remote interpreting services and text telephones (TTY) or text messaging, when communications are difficult with standard telephones. In other words, you have options that enhance opportunities to work and help you accommodate to a job, once you secure it.

Building Confidence

At times every teen feels a lack of confidence or feels different. Join the club. But you may believe life is more difficult because you have a speech and language challenge. Perhaps it is in some ways. But difficulty speaking does not have to define you or make you feel shyer or less capable or able to succeed. As Eleanor Roosevelt, social activist, author, and wife of President Franklin Roosevelt once said, "No one can make you feel inferior without your consent."[5] Make it your business to never consent.

As mentioned earlier, one thing you can do to build confidence is to discover your talents and build on them. Sports, music, art, dancing, volunteering. Finding what you enjoy and do best can be a big esteem booster.

Another confidence builder involves taking care of yourself. Organize your bedroom and school supplies, prepare nutritious lunches, keep your clothes clean and wrinkle-free. If you are healthy and well-groomed, you will feel better about yourself. And that job you found? Nothing like successful employment outside the home and bringing home a paycheck to build confidence.

Forget rejections at school or by certain individuals. Your opinion counts. You can be assertive and make yourself understood. You can succeed in a different

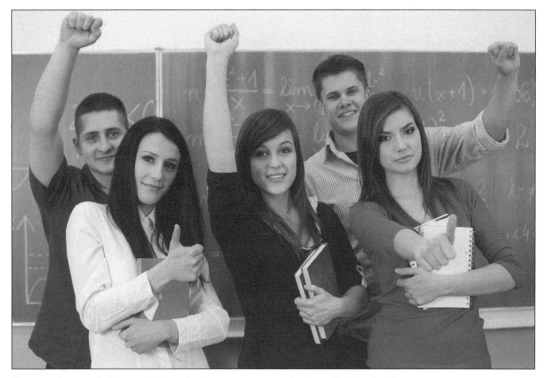

No one is good at everything, but everyone can be good at trying!

environment with different people. There may be a few bumps in the road—with communications or generally. But you can succeed anywhere you choose.

Resources

Organizations/Websites

Americans with Disabilities Act home page
www.ada.gov
ADA Infoline: 800-514-0301 (voice); 800-514-0383 (TTY)
Offers the latest information about the federal law that ensures workplace and general rights for people with disabilities, including communication disorders.

U.S. Department of Justice
Civil Rights Division
950 Pennsylvania Avenue NW
Disability Rights Section-NYAV
Washington, DC 20530
www.justice.gov
800-514-0301 (voice); 800-514-0383 (TTY)
Place to contact if we feel we are experiencing job discrimination.

Go Ask Alice!
goaskalice.columbia.edu
Internet social and health resource site that answers anonymous questions about health and well-being. No topic is off-limits; responses cover everything from sex education and relationship issues to general health. Responses come from a team of health care information and research specialists from Columbia University.

Office of Adolescent Health
Department of Health and Human Services
1101 Wootton Parkway, Suite 700
Rockville, MD 20852
www.hhs.gov
Federal program with contacts and a website dedicated to improving the health and well-being of adolescents that covers varied topics, such as self-esteem, talking with parents, and dating.

ShyKids
www.shykids.com

Website written by former shy students and their parents that tackles aspects of shyness from building confidence to social anxiety.

Speechville Express
www.speechville.com
Site for anyone who struggles with communication challenges that includes information, products and resources, and online support services.

Glossary

accent: the distinctive way people speak the same language

agnosia: a condition whereby someone can understand words but cannot pick up other clues that go along with speaking, such as gestures or tone

aphasia: a language disorder whereby someone is unable to understand or express the spoken word or a combination of the two

apraxia: a motor speech disorder resulting from a neurological, or brain, condition that interferes with muscle control involved in speech production

articulation: how speech sounds are made

Asperger's syndrome: the mildest form of autism that interferes with language development and results in awkward social skills and communication that appears flat, rote, or off in some way

audiologist: specialist trained in preventing, diagnosing, and identifying hearing loss not connected to another medical condition or treatment

autism spectrum disorder: the range of autism signs involving language and social skills that can be mild to severe

bilingual: the ability to speak fluently and understand more than one language

blocking: when air from the lungs gets stuck, rather than flows through the mouth, making talking fluently impossible

bouncing: speaking pattern of repeating sounds and syllables, seemingly stuck on them

chromosomes: the material in genes that carries traits inherited from both parents

cochlear implant: surgery for nerve hearing loss that seeks to convert sound waves to electrical pulses in order to stimulate the nerve and heighten perceptions

concussion: formal term for traumatic brain injury from a jolt or blow to the head that is hard enough to alter the way the brain usually works

conductive hearing loss: when hearing is reduced due to blockage anywhere along the path sound waves take through the outer, middle, and inner ear to the brain

coteaching: learning situation that involves two teachers: one to teach academic subjects, and a special education teacher to support specific learning goals for students with designated adaptations

cyberbullying: when an individual posts nasty or untrue messages about someone else

decibels: units of measurement for sounds and noise

delayed language: when young children progress slowly in their language development

development: process of gaining new skills that build on formerly learned ones

disfluency: problem with fluency of spoken language

dominant language: the language someone uses to feel comfortable speaking and to learn best

dopamine: chemical in the brain that affects motor control over speaking

dyslexia: a language-based learning disability that results in lifelong problems with language, including spelling, reading, and writing

dysphonia: inability to speak, usually caused by strained vocal cords due to overuse

eardrum: the membrane, also called the tympanic membrane, that allows sound waves to pass into the middle ear

expressive aphasia: impairment of the ability to communicate messages

expressive language: ability to relate information through words, symbols, and gestures

fluency: rhythm of word flow

global aphasia: brain impairment that contributes to aphasia of both receptive and expressive language

glottal attack: more often, the hard, abrupt eruption when someone begins to speak, although some speakers may have soft glottal attacks and begin speaking slowly

inner ear: innermost part of the auditory system that contains fluid that moves delicate hairs and translates sound waves into nerve impulses in the brain

internship: a job situation whereby someone offers a given amount of time and labor in exchange for professional supervision

language: set of communication rules that are shared by a social group that permits members to exchange ideas, emotions, or thoughts

language disorder: difficulty understanding and using spoken, written, or symbolic language

laryngitis: a common cause of hoarseness from illness, allergies, or exposure to harsh chemicals that can result in complete loss of voice

larynx: passageway between the base of the tongue and top of the trachea, or passageway to the lungs

learning disability: brain disorder that influences learning

lisp: speech production that substitutes letters *s* and *z* with the sounds for *th*

lobes: main sections of the brain that are responsible for different body functions

middle ear: part of the hearing system that contains three tiny vibrating bones that pulsate and send sound waves into the inner ear and toward the brain

milestones: specific steps doctors and educators observe to determine whether someone is developing in a typical manner

neurologist: doctor who deals with the nervous system, including the brain

oral cavity: upper end of the vocal tract that contains the tongue, pharynx, hard and soft palates, lips, and jaw

otolaryngologist: doctor concerned with ears, nose, and throat

otosclerosis: a condition whereby a growth develops around middle ear bones during teen years, inhibiting movement of sound waves

phonological processes: atypical sound patterns

prolongation: speaking pattern of holding onto a sound for longer than necessary for regular speech

receptive aphasia: impairment in the ability to understand incoming messages

receptive language: ability to understand words, symbols, and gestures

repetition: speaking pattern of repeating the same syllable several times before being able to move onto another syllable or word

resonance: voice quality that results from how air passes through various chambers and cavities to make sounds

resource class: version of special education study hall, where a special education teacher who understands study strategies helps students plan and use time better

rewiring: when one side of the brain takes over tasks usually handled by the other, such as with stuttering

shadowing: an opportunity for someone to experience what is involved in a given job by following a professional who does that job through their day

social pragmatics: the cultural and social aspects of getting along that most people usually learn automatically as they mature

speech: how we communicate verbally

speech and language pathologist: specialist who helps clients evaluate and improve their ability to convey meaningful messages

speech sound disorders: when language is difficult to understand during conversation due to substituting, replacing, distorting, or leaving off sounds and words

stroke: when brain injury interrupts blood flow in the brain, which can interfere with communication

sudden sensorineural hearing loss: a type of hearing loss that appears without warning and arises from damage to the auditory nerve

supported education: learning situation that adds a special education aide in the classroom to help answer individual questions, reinforce material, and provide accommodations, such as extra time for tests

tinnitus: ringing in the ear that reduces the ability to hear

trachea: passageway to the lungs

vocal folds: two bands of smooth muscle tissue that line the larynx

vocal fry: way of speaking with low, raspy sounds that has gained popularity among teen females

vocal tract: source of speech production that includes vocal cords and oral and nasal cavities

voice: how breathing works with vocal folds to produce sound

Notes

Introduction

1. U.S. Department of Education, Office of Special Education Programs, "Indicator 9. Children and Youth with Disabilities," in *Annual Report to Congress on the Implementation of the Individuals with Disabilities Education Act*, table A9-9, nces.ed.gov/programs/coe/indicator_cgg.asp (accessed March 27, 2013).
2. National Dissemination Center for Children with Disabilities, "Speech-Language Impairments" (Disability Fact Sheet 11), January 2011, p. 2.
3. National Institute on Deafness and Other Communication Disorders, "Stuttering," www.nidcd.nih.gov/health/voice/pages/stutter.aspx (accessed March 29, 2013).

a. "VP Joe Biden, Former Stutterer, Connects Speech Excellence to Movie," *Examiner.com*, September 8, 2012, www.examiner.com/article/vp-joe-biden-former-stutterer-connects-speech-excellence-to-movie (accessed November 25, 2013).

Chapter 1

1. National Dissemination Center for Children with Disabilities, "Speech & Language Impairments" (Disability Fact Sheet 11), January 2011, p. 1.
2. Lu Ann Franklin, "Fluent Connection Children's Speech Therapy Keyed into Classroom Experience," *Chicago Tribune*, March 5, 2000, 18.14.
3. Ermon Vandy, interview with author, June 7, 2013.

a. Big Think Editors, "Does Language Change How We Think? Ask the Hyper-Polyglot Teen Who Speaks 20 of Them," Big Think, June 6, 2013, bigthink.com/big-think-tv/does-language-change-how-we-think-ask-the-hyper-polyglot-teen-who-speaks-20-of-them (accessed June 13, 2013).
b. Walter Hickey, "22 Maps That Show How Americans Speak English Totally Differently from Each Other," *Business Insider*, June 5, 2013, www.businessinsider.com/22-maps-that-show-the-deepest-linguistic-conflicts-in-america-2013-6?op=1 (accessed June 5, 2013).
c. Jesse Richardson-Jones, "Speaking Up: Gene Tells Human Tale," Facts on File, December 2009, www.2facts.com/PrintPage.aspx?PIN=s1700159 (accessed May 29, 2013).
d. Joanne Hein, interview with author, March 14, 2013.
e. American Speech-Language-Hearing Association, "Talking with Your Audiologist or SLP: Getting the Most from Your Visit," www.asha.org/public/talkingwithaudorslp.htm (accessed May 7, 2013).

Chapter 2

1. The Stuttering Foundation, "FAQ," www.stutteringhelp.org/faq (accessed May 10, 2013).
2. The Stuttering Foundation, "FAQ."
3. Suzi Shulman, speech therapist, interview with author, August 8, 2013.
4. Barry Harbaugh, "A History of Stuttering in the Movies," Slate.com, December 9, 2010, www.slate.com/articles/arts/culturebox/2010/12/a_history_of_stuttering_in_the_movies.html.
5. Andrew Comstock, *A System of Elocution, with Special Reference to Gesture, Treatment of Stammering and Defective Articulation*, 18th ed. (Philadelphia: E.H. Butler & Company, 1855), 31–33.
6. Joseph Brownstein, "Stuttering May Have Genetic Roots, Study Suggests," *ABC News*, February 11, 2010, abcnews.go.com/Health/MindMoodNews/stuttering-genes-lead-speech-condition/story?id=9802285 (accessed June 13, 2013).
7. Wynne Parry, "Brain Changes in Those Who Stutter Involve More Than Speech," the Stuttering Foundation, August 16, 2011, www.stutteringhelp.org/brain-changes-those-who-stutter-involve-more-speech (accessed May 10, 2013).
8. Rachel Duginske and Lisa LaSalle, "Auditory Processing Skills and Abilities in Children Who Stutter," ASHA 2008, Technical session, 1559, pp. 12–13.
9. "The King's Speech and Stuttering: Interview with Thomas David Kehoe," *Sensory Smart Parent Blog*, January 14, 2011, sensorysmartparent.wordpress.com/tag/auditory-processing-stuttering (accessed June 14, 2013).
10. Marlo Thomas, *The Right Words at the Right Time* (New York: Atria Books, 2002), 317.
11. Craig Coleman, "Ask the Expert," *Family Voices*, Second Quarter, 2013, p. 2.
12. Stuttering Project at the University of Iowa, "Frequently Asked Questions about Stuttering," clas.uiowa.edu/comsci/research/stuttering-research-lab/faqs (accessed May 13, 2013).
13. Peter Ramig, "Don't Ever Give Up!" in *Advice to Those Who Stutter* (Memphis, TN: Stuttering Foundation of America, 2008), 46.
14. Kenneth St. Louis, "Cluttering Updated," *ASHA Leader*, November 18, 2003, www.asha.org/Publications/leader/2003/031118/f031118a.htm (accessed June 18, 2013).
15. William Smith, "Fluency Disorders: Stuttering vs Cluttering," Ezine Articles, ezinearticles.com/?Fluency-Disorders:-Stuttering-vs-Clutterin&id=335383 (accessed June 5, 2013).

a. Susannah Parkin, interview with author, June 23, 2013.
b. Autobiographical experience of author, June 5, 2013.
c. Softpedia, "Shane Garcia on *So You Think You Can Dance* Is the Most Amazing Thing You'll See Today" (video), updated February 2013, news.softpedia.com/news/Shane-Garcia-on-So-You-Think-You-Can-Dance-Is-the-Most-Amazing-Thing-You-ll-See-Today-355443.shtml (accessed June 18, 2013).
d. Softpedia, "Shane Garcia."
e. Softpedia, "Shane Garcia."
f. "Lazaro Arbos, American Idol Tryout," *People* video, www.thehollywoodgossip.com/videos/lazaro-arbos-american-idol-audition, January 1, 2013 (accessed June 18, 2013).
g. Kelley Benham, *St. Petersburg Times*, "Sean's Echo," June 1, 2004, accessed May 30, 2013.
h. "Lazaro Arbos, American Idol Tryout."

i. Steve Charing, "'American Idol's' Lazaro Inspires Us All," *Steve Charing OUTspoken* (blog), March 18, 2013, stevecharing.blogspot.com/2013/03/american-idols-lazaro-inspires-us-all .html, (accessed May 30, 2013).

j. Tim Nudd, "Lazaro Arbos Wants to Visit *Glee's* William McKinley High School Next," *People*, April 12, 2013, www.people.com/people/article/0,,20690773,00.html (accessed June 11, 2013).

k. Voon Pang, "The Lazaro Effect," the Stuttering Foundation, May 2, 2013, www.stuttering help.org/blog/lazaro-effect (accessed May10, 2013).

l. Harbaugh,"A History of Stuttering in the Movies."

m. Thomas, *The Right Words*, 317–320.

n. Jacky G., "Winston Churchill's Dentures," *Speech Buddies* (blog), www.speechbuddy.com/ blog/speech-disorders-2/winston-churchills-dentures/ (accessed August 14, 2013).

o. Greg Wilson, "Singing and Stuttering: What We Know," the Stuttering Foundation, www.stutteringhelp.org/content/singing-and-stuttering-what-we-know-0 (accessed May 13, 2013).

p. Dorvan Breitenfeldt, "Managing Your Stuttering Versus Your Stuttering Managing You," in *Advice to Those Who Stutter* (Memphis, TN: The Stuttering Foundation of America, 2008), 1.

q. Lil JaXe: Official Site liljaxe.com (accessed November 27, 2013).

r. The Stuttering Foundation, "Famous People Who Stutter," www.stutteringhelp.org/famous -people-who-stutter, p. 107.

Chapter 3

1. National Institute of Deafness and Other Communication Disorders, "Statistics on Voice, Speech, and Language" (NIDCD Health Information), www.nidcd.nih.gov/health/statistics/ pages/vsl.aspx (accessed June 26, 2013).

2. J. L. Preston, M. Hull, and M. L. Edwards, "Preschool Speech Error Patterns Predict Articulation and Phonological Awareness Outcomes in Children with Histories of Speech Sound Disorders," *American Journal of Speech and Language Pathology* 22, no. 2 (May 2013): 173–84, EPub, November 26, 2012, www.ncbi.nlm.nih.gov/pubmed/23184137 (accessed June 26, 2013).

3. Suzi Shulman, interview with author, June 24, 2013.

4. Daniel Boone and Elena Plante, *Human Communication and Its Disorders*, 2nd ed. (Englewood Cliffs, NJ: Prentice Hall, 1993), 259.

5. Christy Cook, interview with author, April 5, 2013.

6. Cook, interview.

a. ShyKids.com, "About shykids," www.shykids.com/aboutshykids.htm (accessed July 1, 2013).

b. M, "Bothered," posted on the page "Letters to a Speech-Language Pathologist about Lisping," Speech-Language-Therapy.com, updated on Friday, March 2, 2012, www.speech -language-therapy.com/index.php?option=com_content&view=article&id=91:letters&catid =11:admin, p. 4 (accessed April 22, 2014).

c. Caroline Bowern, "Beyond Lisping—Code Switching and Gay Speech Styles," speech -language-therapy.com/index.php?option=com_content&view=article&id=62:code&catid= 11:admin&Itemid=117 (accessed June 24, 2013).

d. Jeanne Buesser, *He Talks Funny* (Bloomington, IN: AuthorHouse, 2011).

e. Trent Reedy, *Words in the Dust* (New York: Arthur Levine Books, 2011).

f. Roxanne Swentzell, interview with author, July 6, 2013.

g. Roxanne Swentzell, "Poems to My Sculptures," About Roxanne, www.swentzell.com/mainpages/aboutRox.html (accessed July 8, 2012).

h. Anne Stein, "New Tools to Help Kids with Speech Disorders," *Chicago Tribune*, May 15, 2011, p. 6.21, available at articles.chicagotribune.com/2011-04-13/a-z/sc-health-0413-speech-buddies-20110413_1_disorders-speech-pathology-and-audiology-tongue. (accessed June 23, 2013).

i. Matt Alden, "Bullying," Matt's Hideout, www.matts-hideout.co.uk.

j. Adrienne Van Der Valk, "There Are No Bullies: Just Children Who Bully—and You Can Help Them," *Teaching Tolerance* no. 45 (Fall 2013): 38–41.

Chapter 4

1. Daniel Boone and Elena Plante, *Human Communication and Its Disorders*, 2nd ed. (Englewood Cliffs, NJ: Prentice Hall, 1993), 305.

2. Katherine Hobson, "The Vocal Cord Injury Affecting Adele," *Health Blog* (*Wall Street Journal*), October 7, 2011, blogs.wsj.com/health/2011/10/07/the-vocal-cord-injury-affecting-adele/ (accessed December 4, 2013).

3. American Academy of Otolaryngology, "Fact Sheet: Nodules, Polyps, and Cysts," entnet.org/HealthInformation/nodPolypCysts.cfm (accessed May 6, 2013).

a. Adapted from Boone, *Human Communication and Its Disorders*, 286–87.

b. Stephanie Zacharias, et al., "Teachers' Perceptions of Adolescent Females with Voice Disorders," *Language, Speech, and Hearing Services in Schools* 44 (April 2013): 174–82, udini.proquest.com/view/middle-and-high-school-teachers-goid:866208905 (accessed May 2013).

c. Fred Bronson, "Q & A: David Archuleta of 'American Idol,'" *Billboard*, May 6, 2008, December 4, 2013.

d. Angelica, "Cords of Love: David Archuleta," *Voice*, August 4, 2010.

e. Angelica, "Cords of Love."

f. Patrick Healy, "The Smoke Has Cleared: Time to Rest," *New York Times*, July 3, 2013, C1.

g. Hobson, "The Vocal Cord Injury Affecting Adele."

h. American Academy of Otolaryngology, "Fact Sheet: Nodules, Polyps, and Cysts," www.entnet.org/HealthInformation/nodPolypCysts.cfm (accessed May 6, 2013).

i. Kyle Anderson, "John Mayer Announces First Pot Throat Surgery Tour," *Entertainment Weekly*, March 22, 2013, music-mix.ew.com/2013.03/22/john-mayer-new-tour-2013 (accessed July 8, 2013).

j. Faith Sallie, "Burned Out on the 'Fry,'" *CBS News*, September 8, 2013, www.cbsnews.com/2102-3445_162-57601876.html (accessed September 8, 2013).

k. Katy Steinmetz, "Get Your Creak On: Is 'Vocal Fry' a Female Fad?" *Time.com*, December 15, 2011, healthland.time.com/2011/12/15/get-your-creak-on-is-vocal-fry-a-female-fad/ (accessed September 8, 2013).

Chapter 5

1. Oliver Sacks, "The President's Speech," in *The Man Who Mistook His Wife for a Hat* (New York: Harper & Row, 1985), 80–91).
2. Sacks, "The President's Speech," 83–84.
3. National Dissemination Center for Children with Disabilities, "Speech & Language Impairments" (Disability Fact Sheet 11), January 2011, p. 3, nichcy.org (accessed March 3, 2013); from Encyclopedia of Nursing & Allied Health, "Language Disorders," www.enotes.com/nursing-encyclopedia/language-disorders.
4. National Institute on Deafness and Other Communication Disorders Health Information, "Statistics on Voice, Speech, and Language," www.nidcd.nih.gov/health/statistics/pages/vsl.aspx, p. 3 (accessed June 26, 2013).
5. Marat Moore, "Teens at Risk: 'We're on the Edge of an Epidemic,'" *ASHA Leader*, September 21, 2010, www.asha.org/Publications/leader/2010/100921/Teens-at-Risk.htm (accessed July 24, 2013).
6. Daniel Boone and Elena Plante, *Human Communications and Its Disorders*, 2nd ed. (Englewood Cliffs, NJ: Prentice Hall, 1993), 103.
7. Veronica Getskow and Dee Konczal, *Kids with Special Needs* (Santa Barbara, CA: Learning Works, 1996), 98.
8. American Speech-Language-Hearing Association (ASHA), "Incidence and Prevalence of Communication Disorders and Hearing Loss in Children—2008 Edition," www.asha.org/Research/reports/children, p. 2 (accessed August 10, 2012).
9. ASHA, "Incidence and Prevalence," 2.
10. ASHA, "Language-Based Learning Disabilities," www.asha.org/public/speech/disorders/lbld.htm, p. 1 (accessed July 11, 2013).
11. National Institute of Neurological Disorders and Stroke, "Autism Fact Sheet," www.ninds.nih.gov/disorders/autism/detail_autism.htm (accessed May 24, 2013).
12. Marlene Targ Brill, *Keys to Parenting the Child with Autism* (Hauppauge, NY: Barron's Educational Series, 2001), 29.

---

a. Katy, interview with author, June 6, 2013.
b. Nicholas Bakalar, "Obesity and Hearing Loss," *New York Times*, June 25, 2013, D6.
c. Karena Weil, counselor at the Hearing and Speech Center of North California, interview with author, June 14, 2013.
d. Joyce Cohen, "Want a Better Listener? Protect Those Ears," *New York Times*, Science, March 2, 2010, D6, p. 1, www.nytimes.com/2010/03/02/health/02baby.html?_r=0 (accessed November 1, 2012).
e. News Center: The University of Utah, "Drivers on Cell Phones Are as Bad as Drunks," June 29, 2006, www.unews.utah.edu/old/p/062206-1.html (accessed August 27, 2013).
f. Sam Sagmiller, "Famous Dyslexics and Famous People with Learning Disabilities," Dyslexia My Life, dyslexiamylife.org/who_els.html, pp. 1–3 (accessed July 16, 2013).
g. Stuart Kaufman, interview with author, July 22, 2013.
h. Adapted from Sam Sagmiller, "Dyslexia Helpful Tips," Dyslexia My Life, www.dyslexiamylife.org, p. 4 (accessed July 16, 2013).
i. John, interview with author, February 4, 2001.

j.   "Miss Montana Alexis Wineman to Become First Autistic Miss America Contestant," *FoxNews .com*, January 10, 2013, www.foxnews.com/entertainment/2013/01/10/miss-montana-alexis -wineman-to-become-first-autistic-miss-america-contestant/ (accessed August 2, 2013).

k.   Temple Grandin, *Thinking in Pictures* (New York: Doubleday, 1995), 19–20.

l.   Temple Grandin's website, www.templegrandin.com (accessed July 22, 2013).

m.   Temple Grandin' website, www.templegrandin.com, from *Emergence: Labeled Autistic* (New York: Warner Books, 1996) (accessed July 22, 2013).

Chapter 6

1.   American Medical Association, *Complete Medical Guide* (New York: Random House, 2003), 1234.

2.   Brain Injury Association of America (BIAA), "Living with Brain Injury," 2013, www .biausa.org/living-with-brain-injury.htm, p. 1 (accessed August 5, 2013).

3.   BIAA, "BIAA Statement on Congresswoman Giffords," January 10, 2011, www.biausa.org/ announcements/biaa-statement-on-congresswoman-giffords (accessed May 8, 2013).

4.   BIAA, "Living with Brain Injury," 2.

5.   Aphasia and Neurolinguistics Laboratory, "Finding the Right Words," Northwestern School of Communication, Fall 2013, www.northwestern.edu/magazine/fall2013/campuslife/ finding-the-right-words.html, p. 15.

6.   Aphasia and Neurolinguistics Laboratory, "Finding the Right Words," 15.

7.   Oliver Sacks, *The Mind's Eye* (New York: Alfred A. Knopf, 2010), 34–35.

8.   National Institute on Deafness and Other Communication Disorders, "Statistics on Voice, Speech, and Language," www.nidcd.nih.gov/health/statistics/pages/vsl.aspx (accessed June 26, 2013).

9.   National Center for Injury Prevention and Control, "10 Leading Causes of Violence-Related Injury Deaths, U.S. 2010, All Races, Both Sexes," Centers for Disease Control and Prevention, webappa.cdc.gov/cgi-bin/broker.ex (accessed December 4, 2010); Centers for Disease Control and Prevention (CDC), "Teen Drivers: Fact Sheet," www.cdc.gov/Motorvehicle safety/teen_drivers/teendrivers_factsheet.html, p. 1 (accessed July 29, 2013).

10.   CDC, "Teen Drivers," 2.

11.   ThinkFirst, "Fast Facts: Roller Sports Safety," in *Newsletter of the Calgary Injury Prevention Coalition*, p. 200, www.thinkfirst.org; also from www.safekids.org/tier3_cd.cfm?contact_ item_id=1211&folder_id-540 (accessed August 5, 2013).

12.   ThinkFirst, "Fast Facts," 3.

13.   Hamilton Cain, "Sports Medicine," *New York Times Magazine*, September 14, 2008, 26.

14.   BIAA, "Brain Injury: The Teenage Years, Understanding and Preventing Teenage Brain Injury," www.biausa.org, p. 8 (accessed May 8, 2013).

15.   Ken Belson, "Concussion Study Makes Case to Curb Practice Hits," *New York Times*, July 26, 2013, Sports, B11.

16.   Bill Pennington, "New Rule at NFL's Camps: No Tackling. It's Just Practice," *New York Times*, August 1, 2013, B13.

a.   Shannon Thomas, interview with author, May 5, 2013.

b.   BrainlineKids, "Acquired Brain Injury: Teens Talking to Teens: Sabrina" (ten-minute video of teen describing her TBI and recovery), Brainline, www.brainline.org/content/multimedia .php?id=901 (accessed December 4, 2013).

c. BIAA, "Brain Injury Facts: About Brain Injury," www.biausa.org (go to "Brain Injury FAQs") (accessed May 8, 2013).

d. Kristen's story is adapted from an interview conducted for Aphasia and Neurolinguistics Laboratory, "Finding the Right Words," *Northwestern*, www.northwestern.edu/magazine/fall2013/campuslife/finding-the-right-words.html (accessed May 15 2013).

e. Aphasia and Neurolinguistics Laboratory, comm.soc.northwestern.edu/aphasia (accessed May 15, 2013).

f. Kerry Lester, "Illinois Senator Mark Kirk Pen/Pals with 11-year-old Stroke Victim, Jackson Cunningham," September 18, 2013, *HuffPost Good News*, December 15, 2013, www.huffingtonpost.com/2013/09/18/mark-kirk-pen-pal_n_3950858.html (accessed December 15, 2013).

g. Mark Emmons, "Gilroy Teen's Traumatic Brain Injury Affects Entire Family," *San Jose Mercury News*, January 14, 2013, www.mercurynews.com/ci_22370885/gilroy-teens-traumatic-brain-injury-affects-entire-family (accessed December 15, 2013).

h. Autobiographical experience of author, September 29, 2013.

Chapter 7

1. National Center for Education Statistics, "NAEP Data Explorer," nces.ed.gov/nations reportcard/naepdata/report.aspx?app=NDE&p=1-MAT-2-20113%2c20093%2c20073%2c20053%2c20033%2c20003%2c20002%2c19963%2c19962%2c19922%2c19902-MRPCM-SDRACE-NT-RP_RP-Y_J-0-0-5 (accessed December 5, 2013).

2. United Nations Educational Scientific and Cultural Organization (UNESCO), "Languages in Education," portal.unesco.org/education/en/ev.php-URL_ID=28301&URL_DO-DO_TOPIC&U, p. 1 (accessed July 16, 2013).

3. American Speech-Language-Hearing Association (ASHA), "The Advantages of Being Bilingual," www.asha.org/public/speech/development/The-Advantages-of-Being-Bilingual/, p. 1 (accessed January 10, 2013).

4. Public Broadcasting System, *In the Mix*, "Teen Immigrants: Five American Stories: Myths and Facts," www.pbs.org/inthemix/shows/show_teen_immigrants3.html, p. 2 (accessed August 6, 2013).

5. Mayra Daniel, "Young ELLs at K–2nd Are Biliterate: Let's Understand What They Are Doing and Help Them Enjoy the Process," Northern Illinois University Summer Conference, 2009, pp. 1–2.

6. Susan Boswell and Carol Polovoy, "Bridging Cultures in the Schools," *ASHA Leader*, September 25, 2007, www.asha.org/Publications/leader/2007/070925/070925a.htm, p. 1 (accessed August 7, 2012).

7. Vernon McClean, "How Racism Is Embedded in the Fabric of Language," *New York Times*, January 24, 1988.

8. "Native American Awareness for Educators and School Psychologists," www.minotstateu.edu/schpsych/ndasp/Native.htm referred from G. S. Mosley-Howard, "Best Practices in Considering the Role of Culture," in *Best Practices in School Psychology*, ed. A. Thomas and J. Grimes, 337–345 (Washington, DC: National Association of School Psychologists. *Best Practices in Considering the Role of Culture*, 1995) (accessed September 5, 2013).

9. ASHA, "Accent Modification," www.asha.org/public/speech/development/accent_mod.htm?LangType=1033, p. 1 (accessed June 24, 2013).

10. Richard Perez-Pena, "Providing a Path from Foreign Lips to American Ears," *New York Times*, August 29, 2013, A17.

11. ASHA, "Social Pragmatics Defined," www.asha.org/policy/RP1982-00125/ (accessed June 25, 2013).

---

a. Public Broadcasting System, "Teen Immigrants: Five American Stories: Myths and Facts," on *In the Mix*, www.pbs.org/inthemix/shows/show_teen_immigrants5.html, p. 1–2 (accessed August 6, 2013).

b. From teen transcript interview, Public Broadcasting System, "Teen Immigrants," p. 2.

c. Sonia Sotomayor, *My Beloved World* (New York: Alfred A. Knopf, 2009), 134.

d. Sotomayor, *My Beloved World*, 157.

e. From teen transcript interview, "Meet Young Immigrants," Scholastic.com, teacher.scholastic.com/activities/immigration/young_immigrants/gabriella.htm (accessed April 22, 2014).

f. Maria Jarmel and Ken Schneider, "About the Film," *Speaking in Tongues*, Patchwork Films, speakingintonguesfilm.info/the-film/about-the-film/ (accessed August 13, 2013).

g. Dr. Emory Campbell, *Gullah Cultural Legacies*, 3rd ed. (South Carolina: Gullah Heritage Consulting Services, 2006), www.gullaheritage.com, Book web page, p. 1.

h. Kimberly Fujioka, "The Talking Stick: An American Indian Tradition in the ESL Classroom," *Internet TESL Journal*, iteslj.org/Techniques/Fujioka-TalkingStick.html (accessed September 6, 2013); and Arlene Hirschfelder and Yvonne Beamer, *Native American Today* (Englewood, CO: Teacher Ideas Press, 2000), xv.

i. From Mike Vuolo, "Lexicon Valley: Is Black English a Dialect or a Language?" (podcast), *Slate*, February 27, 2013, www.slate.com/articles/podcasts/lexicon_valley/2012/02/lexicon_valley_is_black_english_a_dialect_or_a_language_.html (accessed August 15, 2013).

j. Suzi Shulman, speech therapist, interview with author, August 5, 2013.

k. Claudia Dreifus, "Defecting to Great Scientific Success," *New York Times*, July 23, 2013, D2.

l. UNESCO, "Education-1.Languages and Writing," portal.unesco.org, p. 1 (accessed August 16, 2013).

m. Farborz Rahnamon, "History of Persian or Parsi Language," www.iranchamber.com (accessed April 14, 2013).

n. Boswell and Polovoy, "Bridging Cultures in Schools," 3.

Chapter 8

1. National Dissemination Center for Children with Disabilities (NICHCY), "Assistive Technology Act," Resources updated, April 2013: Findings and Purposes, Assistive Technology Act of 1998, Finding 3, nichcy.org/laws/ata, p. 1 (accessed August 9, 2013).

2. Amanda Lenhart et al., "Teen and Mobile Phones," Pew Research Internet Project, April 20, 2012, www.pewinternet.org/Reports/2010/Teens-and-Mobile-Phones.aspx (accessed August 27, 2013).

3. Joanna Brenner, "Pew Internet: Teens," Pew Research Center's Internet and American Life Projects, May 21, 2012, www.pewresearch.org/search/facebook+teens/?site=pewinternet (accessed August 27, 2013).

4. Pew Research Center's Internet & American Life Project, "Teens Fact Sheet," May 21, 2012, pewinternet.org/Commentary/2012/April/Pew-Internet-Teens.aspx, pp. 1–3 (accessed August 27, 2013).

5. Pew Research Center's Internet & American Life Project, "Teens Fact Sheet," 3.

6. Pew Internet Parent/Teen Privacy Survey, "Teens on Facebook: What They Share with Friends," Pew Research Center, September 30, 2012, www.pewresearch.org/2013/05/21/teens-on-facebook (accessed August 27, 2013).

7. Mary Madden et al., "Teens, Social Media, and Privacy," Pew Research Internet Project, www.pewinternet.org/Reports/2013/Teens-Social-Media-And-Privacy.aspx (accessed August 27, 2013).

8. Sharon Hurley Hall, "Problems with Social Networking and Teens," Life 123, www.life123.com/parenting/tweens-teens/social-networking/issues-with-teens-and-social-networking.shtml (accessed August 30, 2013).

9. Hall, "Problems."

10. Suzi Shulman, speech therapist, interview with author, August 8, 2013.

11. Christy Cook, speech therapist, interview with author, February 10, 2013.

12. NICHCY "Assistive Technology Act," 2.

13. Alex Soojung-Kin Pang, "Email Is Killing Us: Reclaim Your Mind from Technology," Salon.com, August 17, 2013, www.salon.com/2013/08/17/reclaim_your_mind_from_technology (accessed August 23, 2013), excerpted from *The Distraction Addiction: Getting the Information You Need and the Communication You Want without Enraging Your Family, Annoying Your Colleagues, and Destroying Your Soul* (New York: Little, Brown, 2013).

14. Amanda Lenhart, "Teens and Technology: Communication Choices," Pew Research Center, July 27, 2005, www.pewinternet.org/2012/03/19/communication-choices (accessed October 10, 2013).

15. Jennifer Weigel, "Friends Are Priceless, but Often Undervalued," *Chicago Tribune*, Section 6, August 25, 2013, NS.

16. Lee Rainie, Amanda Lenhart, and Aaron Smith, "The Tone of Life on Social Networking Sites," Pew Research Center's Internet & American Life Project, www.pewinternet.org/Reports/2012/Social-networking-climate.aspx (accessed August 27, 2012).

17. National Bullying Prevent Center, Teens against Bullying home page, www.pacerteensagainstbullying.org (accessed August 6, 2013).

18. Sameer Hinduja, "Teens and Technology, School District Policy Issues, 2012–2013," Cyberbullying Research Center, September 7, 2012, cyberbullying.us/teens-and-technology-school-district-policy-issues-2012-2013/, pp. 3–4, (accessed August 6, 2013).

19. Soojung-Kim Pang, "Email Is Killing Us."

20. Gary Small and Gigi Vorgan, *Surviving the Technological Alteration of the Modern Mind* (New York: HarperCollins, 2008), 25.

21. Rachel Neuses, "Physically Plugging In Is Causing Us to Mentally Plug Out: The Dangers of Too Much Technology," Student paper, April 19, 2013, p. 4; from Alan Greenblatt, "Impact of Internet on Thinking: Overview," *CQ Researcher: Is the Web Changing the Way We Think?* September 24, 2010, p. 784.

22. Small and Vorgan, *Surviving*, 68.

23. Small and Vorgan, *Surviving*, 68.

---

a. Kaylee, interview with author, August 27, 2013.

b. Nick Bilton, "Fraying at Tethers of Our Phones," *New York Times*, Business Day, September 2, 2013, B5.

c. Carly Fleischman, "About Carly," Carly's Voice, carlysvoice.com/home/aboutcarly (accessed August 7, 2013).

d. Carly Fleischman, "FAQ," Carly's Voice, carlysvoice.com/home/faq, p. 3 (accessed August 7, 2013).

e. Daniel, interview with author, August 27, 2013.

f. Kaylee, interview.

g. Lucy, interview with author, August 27, 2013.

h. MTV, "3 Questions to Ask Yourself about Sexting," A Thin Line, www.athinline.org/facts/sexting (accessed August 6, 2012).

i. Shari, "Texting and Social Networking Creating Big Problems for Teens," Gowanus Lounge, www.gowanuslounge.com/texting-social-networking-creating-big-problems-for-teens (accessed August 30, 2013).

j. Daborah Sontage and Celia Dugger, "The New Immigrant Tide: A Shuttle between Worlds," *New York Times*, July 19, 1998, www.nytimes.com/1998/07/19/nyregion/the-new-immigrant-tide-a-shuttle-between-worlds.html, p. 4.

k. Author, personal experience.

l. Jennifer Ludden, "Teen Texting Sours; Will Social Skills Suffer?" NPR, www.npr.org/templates/story/story.php?storyId=126117811 (accessed August 27, 2013).

Chapter 9

1. Marlene Targ Brill, *Raising Smart Kids for Dummies* (Indianapolis, IN: Wiley, 2003), 100.

2. "Unit 10: Effective Listening Skills," www.asbcentral.com/leadership%20lessons%20pdf/speaking.pdf, p. 2, August 21, 2013.

3. "Unit 10," 1.

4. Brill, *Raising Smart Kids*, 274–75.

5. Eleanor Roosevelt, quoted from *This Is My Story*, www.quotationspage.com/quotes/Eleanor_Roosevelt.

a. Sonia Sotomayor, *My Beloved World* (New York: Alfred A. Knopf, 2013), 111.

b. Sarah Maslin Nir, "Kiss Baby, Smile, Check Phone (Over and Over)," *New York Times*, 1.

c. Arlene Hirschfelder and Yvonne Beamer, *Native American Today* (Englewood, CO: Teacher Ideas Press, 2000), xv.

d. Daniel DeNoon, "Fear of Public Speaking Hardwired," WebMD, April 20, 2006, www.webmd.com/anxiety-panic/guide/20060420/fear-public-speaking, p. 1 (accessed September 9, 2013).

e. Alison Brill, "Back to School Mental Wellness: Tips for Parents/Caregivers of Teens," *Mass Public Health Blog*, September 12, 2013, blog.mass.gov/publichealth/mental-wellness/back-to-school-mental-wellness-tips-for-parentscaregivers-of-teens.

f. Sarah Vans, "What Every Student Needs to Learn," *Teen Ink*, teenink.com/opinion/school_college/article/186431/What-Every-Student-Needs-To-Learn (accessed December 15, 2013).

g. Clint Page, "Top 10 Skills for High School Students," FamilyEducation.com, school.familyeducation.com/skill-builder/college-prep/37653.html?detoured=1 (accessed September 5, 2013).

h. Brill, *Raising Smart Kids*, 259.

i. Composite biography taken from real-life situations.

j. Talia, interview with author, September 27, 2013.

k. U.S. Department of Justice, "A Guide to Disability Rights Laws," ADA.gov, July 2009, www.ada.gov/cguide.htm (accessed September 4, 2013).

l. U.S. Department of Justice, "A Guide to Disability Rights Laws."

Index

accents, 144–46

acid reflux. *See* gastroesophageal reflux disease

active listening, 185

Adele, 69

addiction to technology, 163, *166*, 171, *180*

adolescent behavior, 117

agnosia, 75–76

aggression and brain injury. *See* guns

alcohol and brain injury, 117

American Association of Otolaryngologists, 72

American Medical Association, 106

Americans for Responsible Solutions, *116*

American Society for Testing and Materials, 120

American Speech-Language-Hearing Association, 6n2, *85*, 91, 144, 147; Better Speech and Hearing Month, *86*; certifies professionals, *9*; defining speech disorders, 42, 43

Americans with Disabilities Act, *202*

aphasia, 75, 110–12, *113*

apraxia, *46*

Arbos, Lazarro, *21–23*

Archuleta David, *62*

articulation,

definition of, 42

hearing loss and, 46

Asperger's syndrome, 94, 96, 97

assistive technology, 162–63

attention and technology, 149, 159, 171–72

attention-deficit/hyperactivity disorder (ADHD), 88, *94*, 158, 187, 201

attitude, 186, 187, *194*

audiologist, 9, 12, *179*

autism spectrum disorder, 94–101, *94*, *95*, 148–49, 159, *160*

automobile accidents and brain injury, 117–19

baby talk, 67

Better Hearing and Speech Month, *86*

bilingual education classes, 137–38

bilingual learners, 129–36

birth defects: effecting articulation, 46; effecting voice disorders, 62

Bogart-Bacall syndrome, *64*

body language, 188, 200

Borderline, *137*

Bowen, Caroline, *43*

brain damage, 46, 148–49. *See also* traumatic brain injury

brain function, 107

Brain Injury Association of America, 107, 109, 117

Bullying, 53–54, 169–70, 197

Campbell, Dr. Emory, *142*

Carly's Voice, *160*

cell phones, 165, 168–69, 171, 173, 178, *188*

Center for Neurobiology of Language Recovery, 110

child pornography, sexting as, 170

cleft palate and lip, 46–47, 67

cluttering, 34–38

Clyburn, James, *142*

communication: development of, 1–8; history, *177*; improving, 183–203; relationships and, *165*, 165–166, 183–184; rules of, 148–149; technology and,

155–181. *See also* social pragmatics; speech sound disorders
communication problems: dating with, 197–98; jobs and, 198–203; statistics, 10; time management of, *192–193*
computer addiction, 163
computer apps, 159
computer games, 134, 159
computer-generated voice, *162*
computers, 156, 159, *160*, 161, 168–71
concussion, 125–26
conductive hearing loss, 84
confidence building, 86, *191*, *194*, 196, 197, 203–4
Cook, Christine, 50–51, 52, 158–59
Coughlin, Tom, 125
Crawford, Matthias, *157*
cul de sac resonance, 67
Cunningham, Jackson, *114*
cyberbullying, 169–70
Cyberbullying Research Center, 170
cysts, 69

dating, 197–98
decongestant warning, *63*
Demosthenes, 52
disabilities and technology, 159–64
The Distraction Addiction, 163, 171
dominant language, 130
driving habits, safe, *118–19*
drugs and brain injury, 117
drug therapy for stuttering, 29
dysarthria, 161–62
dyslexia, *89*, *90*, *91*–94, *198*

ear, parts of, 82–83, *83*
ear tubes, 84
Early Exit Transitional classes, 139
Ebert, Roger, *162*
educational software, 159, 161
electronic devices: for stuttering, 29–30; for hearing loss, 86–87; for language disabilities, 159
electronic communication board, 159

email, *158*, 159, 168–69, 174, *180*
English as a Second Language (ESL), 136. *See also* English Language Learners
English Language Deficient (ELD), 136. *See also* English Language Learners
English Language Learners, 136–39, 161
eye contact, 188

Facebook, 156, *160*, *162*, *167*, 168, *188*
family communication, 165–66, 184. *See also* parents
FamilyEducation.com, *192*
family meeting, 165, 196
Fellius: Dr. Jonathon, 123–24; fiber-optic cables, *177*
fluency: normal, 15–17; problems, 17–38
friends: brain injury and, 108; hearing loss and, 80; language disabilities and, 76; listening to, 184

Garcia, Shane, *19–20*
gastroesophageal reflux disease (GERD), 65–67, 68
gay and lisp, 43
gender and speech challenges, 11
genes: autism and, 97; language and, 7; learning disabilities and, 88; speech-sound disorders and, 46
Giffords, Former Congresswoman Gabby, *116*
glottal attack, 62
Glover, Candice, *142*
Gonzales, Christina Diaz, *137*
grammar learning, 132
gratitude journal, 187
Grandin, Temple, *97–98*, *99*
Gullah, *142*
Guns: hearing loss and, *85*; brain injury and, 115–116

hackers, 163
Hearing and Speech Center of North California, *80*

hearing loss, 9, 45, 46, 52, 79–88, 178, *179*

hearing protection, *81–82*

hearing system, 81–*83*

heartburn. *See* gastroesophageal reflux disease

Hein, Joanne, *13*

Hendricks, Howard, 189

heredity. *See* genes

hoarseness, 63, 66

hyper-polyglot, *2*

Individual Education Program (IEP), 11–13

Individuals with Disabilities Act (IDEA), 11–13

Internet, 156, 173, *175–76*

internship, *201*

interviews, *See* job interview

In the Mix, 130, *131*

Jarmel, Maria, *140*

Jobs: 195–203; interview, 198–200; internships and shadowing, *201*

Katz, Joshua, *3*

Kaufman, Stuart, *90*

Kessler Institute of Traumatic Brain Injury, 123–124

King's Speech, 24

Kirk, Senator Mark, *114*

Language; bias, 140; culture and, 2, 129–30, 136, 140–46; definition, 2, 5–6; learning 1–3, 131, *133–34*, 135–*36*; Papau New Guinea and, 130; politics and, *141*; written, *150–53*

language disorders, 75–101; aphasia as, 110; articulation and, 52; causes and numbers of, 77–101; defining, 75–76; hearing and, 79–88. *See also* aphasia

laryngitis, 63–64

laws, 10–13, 162–63, *202*

learning disabilities, 88–94, 148–49

learning styles, 88

lisp, 42, 43; gay and, 45

listening, 184–189

Logue, Lionel, *24*

long-distance calling, *177*

nonlistening, 185–87, *188*

The Man Who Mistook His Wife for a Hat, 75–76

The Mind's Eye, 112

Matt's Hideout, 53

Mayer, John, 69, *71*

Midler, Bette, *65*

motorcycle accidents, 121. *See* automobile accidents

multitasking, 173–74

myths: about people with speech challenges, 11–13; about people who stutter, 26

National Bullying Prevention Center, 169

National Center for Injury Prevention and Control, 115

National Center for Education Statistics, 129

National Dissemination Center for Children with Disabilities, 77, 155

National Football League, 123, 124

National Institutes of Health, 112, *113*

Native American tradition, 143, *143*, *186*, *189*, 196

networking, 201

nerve loss and hearing, 84–86

nervous system diseases, 70

neurologist, 112

New York Times, *147*

nodules, 69

nonverbal communication, 146–47, 188, 200. *See also* social pragmatics

online privacy, 168–71

online research, 174–75, *175–76*

otolaryngologist, 63, 86

otosclerosis, 84

Pang, Alex, 163
Parents: stuttering and, 32–33; handling, 195–97. *See also* family communication
Pew Research Center, 155–56, 157, 163–64
phonological processes: definition of, 42–43
planning ahead: job interviews and, 198, *199*; new school situations and, *195*; public speaking and, *191*
polyps, 69

Rain Man, 99
reading fluency, *152*
research. *See* online research
receptive language, 77
The Red Umbrella, *137*
Rehabilitation Act of 1973, Section 504, *202*
resonance, 67, 69
Rigal, Emily-Anne, 53
Roberson, Shari, *152*
roller sports and brain injury, 120, *121*

Sacks, Oliver, 75–76, 110, 112
Safe Tackling Program, 125
Schneider, Ken, *140*
self-esteem. *See* confidence building
sensory hearing loss, 84–86
sexting, *170–71*
Shuman, Suzi, 45, *146*, 157–58
Shykids, *42*
Simon, Carly, *27*
singing to communicate, *116*
Skype, *165*, *177*
smoking and voice, 65, 72
Snopes.com, *176*
social interactions and language, 146–50
social networks, 156, *158*, *166*, *167*, *172*, 179–80
social pragmatics, 9, 146–50, 151
Sotomayor, Judge Sonia, *136*, *138*, *185*
Speaking in Tongues, *140*

speech: anatomy of, 7–*8*, 63; anxiety, *189–90*; developing and producing 3–8, 131; emotional problems and, 13, 131, 144, 161; mental disorders and, 12
speech and language pathologist (therapist), 9–10, 60–61, 65, 69, *112*, *116*, 160; changing accents, 144–46; social pragmatics learning, 149, 184; stuttering therapy, 28–29; teaching English Language Learners, 138
Speech Buddies, *51*
speech sound disorders, 41–55; causes, 43–47; defining, 41, 42–43; dysarthria, 161–62; evaluation of, 47; history of, 52; incidence of, 41; managing, *192–95*; therapy for, 47, 50–52
Stewart, James, 69
Stratton, Allan, *137*
stroke, 112, *114*, 115
study habits, improving, *192–95*
stuttering: definition of, 17–20; discovering, 27; electronic devices and, 29–30; reactions to, 30–32, 32–33, 201; school and, 33–34; singing and, *31*; support groups, 30; treatments, 27–32
sudden sensorineural hearing loss, 85–86
Swentzell, Roxanne, *48–49*

talking stick, *143*, *189*, 196
team sports and brain injury, 122–36
technology, 156–181, *180*; attention using, 171–172; educational tool, 172–173; pros and cons, 157–162; reading and, 172–173, 174; relationships with, 165–167
Technology-Related Assistance for Individuals with Disabilities Act of 1988 (Tech Act or Public Law 100–407), 162–163
teletherapy, 30
texting, 168–69, *172*, *188*; addiction, 166, *180*; cons, 163, 164, 173, 174; friends and, *167*

A Thin Line, *170*
ThinkFirst, 108–109, 120
Thomas, Supreme Court Justice Clarence, *142*
Thompson, Cynthia, 110–11
time management, *192–93*
tinnitus, 178
traumatic brain injury (TBI), 106–126 ; recovering from, *109–10*
Turned, Dr. Lorenzo, *142*
Twitter, 157, *160*, 165, *188*

USA Football, 125
United States Department of Education 2010 Report to Congress, 10
United Nations Educational, Scientific and Cultural Organization, 129

valley girl, 141
The View, *186*
Vilcek, Jan, *147*
vocabulary learning, 132, 147

vocal cord lesions, 69, 70
vocal cord paralysis, *62*
vocal folds, 63, 69, 70
vocal fry, *71*
vocational training, 161
voice: care of, 72; misuse, 64–65; quality, 67, 69; smoking and, 65; therapy, 69; whispering, 70–72
voice disorders, 59–72; causes of, 61–63; discovering, 59–61; discrimination and, *61*
voice recognition, 161

water sports and brain injury, 122
weight, *80*
Weil, Karena, *80*
We Stop Hate, *53*
whispering, 70–72
Wikipedia, 175
Wineman, Alexis, *96*
Witt, Paul, *190*, *191*
written language, 150–53, *150*

About the Author

Marlene Targ Brill is an award-winning author of seventy books for readers of all ages. She loves writing about quirky topics, such as *Tooth Tales from Around the World*, a 1998 Children's Choice and 2013 Illinois Reads selection. But she particularly enjoys the detective work involved in researching facts about history, people, and science. Before beginning her writing journey, Brill taught children who had special needs. That's where her interest in speech, language, and communication in general took root. She hung with speech pathologists. She learned what they did and why. And she applied this learning to activities that allowed her students to improve their reading, writing, and speaking. Much of this training helped her decide what might help teen readers of this book. To learn more about Marlene and her books and presentations, check out her website at www .marlenetargbrill.com.